Praise for *Healing from Narcissistic Abuse*

"*Healing from Narcissistic Abuse* will be a valuable contribution not only for professionals, but for anyone seeking to understand themselves and live with greater fulfillment."

—Claudia Campos, PhD, clinical psychologist, sexologist, Trauma-Certified (TIC), founder of Latinas USA

"What sets *Healing from Narcissistic Abuse* apart is not just the extraordinary knowledge behind it, but the presence woven through every page. Grace Being and Claudia Cauterucci bring practical insights and soul-level guidance that lead to real growth and change."

—Jennie Larsen Flaker, Director, Marketing Simplify

"*Healing from Narcissistic Abuse* is not just about surviving narcissistic abuse, but about reclaiming one's own light. This isn't just a book; it's a healing manual for our era."

—Sydney Noelle, yoga master teacher, owner of Noelle Flow, holistic wellness influencer

"Claudia Cauterucci and Grace Being have created a book that arrives exactly when it is needed—offering pathways toward self-love, resilience, and inner peace in these turbulent times. This is more than a book; it is a guide for healing and for reclaiming humanity itself."

—Luisa Montero Diaz, Dharma Teacher & Master Teacher, Insight Meditation Community of Washington

"Claudia Cauterucci is an absolute beacon of wisdom and compassion when it comes to healing in all its forms. Her deep expertise in the human system—and the emotional, psychological, and spiritual ways to effect change—is nothing short of inspiring."

—Dr. Julie Lopez, CEO & founder of Viva Partnership, Originator of the Leaders Loving Life Program

"*Healing from Narcissistic Abuse* carries the uncommon gift of weaving clinical mastery with soul-deep truth, arriving as a steadfast light in a moment of history that needs it most."

—Charles Martinez, MSN, FNP-BC, holistic healer

Healing from Narcissistic Abuse

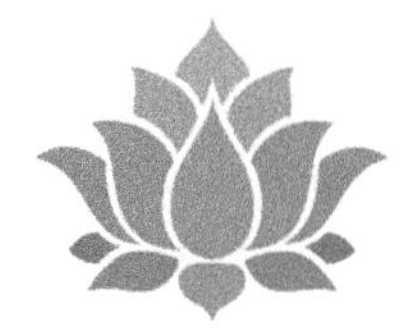

REBUILD FROM RELATIONSHIP TRAUMA

& FIND YOUR LIGHT AGAIN

Grace Being & Claudia Cauterucci, LPC

Hatherleigh Press, Ltd.
62545 State Highway 10, Hobart, NY 13788, USA
hatherleighpress.com

Healing From Narcissistic Abuse

Library of Congress Cataloging-in-Publication Data is available.
ISBN: 978-1-961293-44-1

Cover Design by Carolyn Kasper
Printed in the United States

The authorized representative in the EU for product safety and compliance is Catarina Astrom, Blästorpsvägen 14, 276 35 Borrby, Sweden.
info@hatherleighpress.com

10 9 8 7 6 5 4 3 2 1

CONTENTS

PART III:
Why Are We Attracted to Narcissists?

PART IV:
Recovering From Narcissistic Abuse

AUTHORS' NOTE

NARCISSISTIC ABUSE HAS LONG been a hidden epidemic, but only recently has it started to receive the attention it deserves, given its deep psychological impact. The number of people who end up being victims to narcissistic abuse is mind boggling. Almost everyone has met someone narcissistic throughout their life. It could be at work, a family member, or a romantic partner. The closer the relationship is with the narcissist, the more dramatic and stressful your life is.

Unfortunately, when I ended up a victim of narcissistic abuse, it took me years to realize what was happening. I cannot imagine how many others found themselves falling prey to narcissists, and I believe that raising awareness and educating people about it can help prevent a lot of damage. First and foremost, it's important to acknowledge the fact that narcissistic personality disorder (NPD) is a mental health issue listed in the Diagnostic and Statistical Manual of Mental Disorders, Fifth Edition by the American Psychiatrists Association (DSM-5).

There's a difference between individuals who have narcissistic traits, and those who have a full-blown narcissistic personality disorder. People who suffer from the personality disorder are much more prone to abuse, and they should not be taken lightly. Maintaining a relationship with someone who has a narcissistic personality disorder can make your life a living hell. Knowing what kind of mind games and tactics they use will help you make sense out of what's happening and realize that you are not the one to blame.

Even though it might seem impossible at the moment, I encourage you to hang in there. With the information provided in this book, if you are ready to commit to yourself and do the work, you can transform your pain into something beautiful. Love heals everything. It alchemizes pain into wisdom, fear into courage, and shame into self-acceptance. Cultivating self-love and self-compassion transmutes our emotional wounds, softens their edges, and transforms them into something meaningful. It doesn't erase the past, but it rewrites our relationship to it, helping us grow instead of staying stuck. That's the true power of love: it changes the emotional chemistry of what we carry. And when you learn how to transform your emotional pain into purpose, your inner light will diminish the darkness that had once engulfed your entire being.

But this book is not about them, it's about the people who try to make them happy and end up losing themselves along the way. If you are reading this book and you are one of those people, my heart aches for you, and I sincerely hope that you will find this book useful.

Reading this book will help you feel understood throughout your journey of healing. My story will give you hope and help you change the direction of your life by doing the inner work. When you start reading this book, you embark on a spiritual journey of self-discovery and authenticity. You will find tips, techniques, and life skills to help you understand yourself at a deeper level and support you throughout the recovery process.

As you're reading this book, you will notice that I am narrating my story, as well as explaining the manipulative and abusive techniques used by the narcissist to shed light on their tactics. You'll also notice comments by Claudia Cauterucci, a clinical psychotherapist, throughout the book inside boxes. Claudia shares her insights on the dance between narcissists and their victims, with a focus on the wounded empath. You'll discover that Claudia also has an expertise in making connections between the individual's experience with the narcissist and the collective's experience within narcissistic systems, an approach she calls "the all is in the small and the small is in the all."

Don't be scared to ask for help and seek professional support from a licensed professional if you feel that you need guidance. Healing from narcissistic abuse takes time, patience, a great deal of self-compassion, and self-love. Promise yourself that you will do whatever it takes to heal and break free from the trauma. It's challenging to climb to the top of a mountain, but you know that it's worth the effort when you find yourself at the peak.

When I was writing my book, I put a lot of effort into retrieving painful memories from my mental archive to remember exactly how I used to feel when I was stuck in the abusive relationship. Connecting to my spiritual power gave me the courage and strength to speak my truth in service of others. I am now paying it forward by showing you that you also have the power you need to change the direction of your life.

Lastly, I would like to express my heartfelt gratitude to those who have illuminated my path during my darkest moments and guided me through my journey of healing and spiritual transformation.

First and foremost, I am forever indebted to Tony Macelli, a healer with a compassionate heart, who selflessly devotes his time to helping individuals break free from their emotional wounds. His graceful teachings and exceptional skills have initiated a profound inner transformation within me.

I would like to extend a special thanks to Fr. Gioele Galea, my spiritual mentor, who has illuminated my path with his wisdom and intuition during my spiritual awakenings.

I cannot overlook the immense contributions of Fr. John Vella, my dedicated psychotherapist and Jungian Analyst, whose patience and knowledge guided my deep self-exploration. His assistance in understanding myself, integrating my shadow, and healing fragmented aspects of myself has been invaluable in my journey towards wholeness.

To my parents, Catherine and Mannes, I express my gratitude for their earnest efforts in demonstrating love and instilling good values in me. To my dear sister Rowena, thank you for providing me with resources that helped me on my healing journey.

Lastly, I offer my deepest gratitude to God, Source, my Creator. Your Divine presence and guidance, along with the profound influence of Christ Consciousness, have been the guiding light throughout my journey. I am forever grateful for your grace and unconditional love.

To all these remarkable individuals and God in all Its glory, your presence in my life has been an invaluable gift, and I extend my deepest appreciation for the profound impact you have had on my personal growth and this book.

—Grace

I BELIEVE THAT WE CAN heal through adult bonds of secure attachment. When we feel securely attached, we feel, first and foremost, safe. Safety comes in many forms, and one of them is feeling like our parents, our guides, or the person who knows more than we do—even if it's a few steps more—provides us with information, instructions, and a roadmap, all enveloped in love and patience. This bedrock of safety becomes the launchpad for exploration, expansion, and evolution. In this book, Grace has done this beautifully! You are about to embark on a journey of self-discovery because she has provided the roadmap, the instructions, and the caring resonance you will need to explore deep parts of yourself.

—Claudia

Part I

How It All Started

"The wound is the place where the Light enters you."
—Rumi

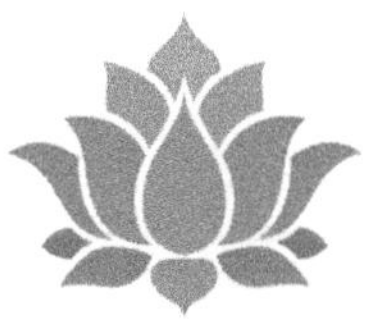

BEFORE WE GET INTO the juicy details and the psychology behind narcissistic personality disorder, I want to share my story with you. As you read it, you may find yourself relating to parts of it, recognizing patterns or behaviors that mirror your own experiences with a narcissist. That's not a coincidence. Narcissists follow strikingly similar patterns. The severity, context, or circumstances may vary, but the core traits are consistent enough to be formally identified and listed as diagnostic criteria in the DSM-5 for narcissistic personality disorder.

When you read my story, you'll see parts of yourself in it, just as I've seen myself in every survivor I've met on this journey. We're connected by shared wounds and experiences.

We may be strangers, but we're also deeply familiar to one another. Through this story, you'll come to know me. I see you. I hear you. I feel you.

Let's begin.

Chapter 1

An Illusion of Bliss

I REMEMBER THE FIRST TIME I saw him, there was something about his energy, something that drew me to him from a distance. I felt a subtle energy, a magnetic pull that was beyond my control. At the time, I was only 24 years old, and I had just got out of a horrible, controlling relationship of four and a half years. I know what you must be thinking, this girl has really terrible taste when it comes to choosing guys, right?! Sounds familiar, perhaps?

The four and a half year relationship, which I had ended just before I met my narcissistic boyfriend, was painful. He had isolated me and made me fight with all my friends, along with my dearest family members. By the age of 22, I didn't have any friends left, and the only person I could hang out with was himself and his family. I was experiencing so much anxiety and stress due to his depressing and possessive personality that my body could not take it anymore, and I developed psychosomatic symptoms. My body felt like it was deteriorating, and I honestly thought that I had a terminal illness.

What Grace is describing here is what I call an "overlap." An overlap occurs when we haven't fully cleaned up on one relationship—it could be from any setting, family, romantic, or work—and move into the next relationship. It's important to take stock, as if we are going through a relational inventory, of what happened, what were the hardest moments, why were they hard, what were your responses, and why. This is best to do in the context of psychotherapy, a support group, or a 12-step group.

Some people define this as a rebound, and yes, a rebound is a form of overlap; a rebound is a way to avoid feelings of loneliness or emptiness and defend against the despair that a severed relationship brings. Most overlaps are about avoidance, defending, and distracting from an intense emptiness or self-hate. The irony is that overlap brings with it what was there before, and possibly makes it worse. The individual "overlapping," in this case, Grace, feels doubly horrible because instead of finding relief in someone new, she found an even deeper abyss of despair.

From a spiritual perspective, we can say that the lesson that needed to be learned is on the table again, but with a more intense request to be seen and heard. Our learnings will call for us at higher and higher volumes if we run from them. We are not here on Earth to be punished; we are here to learn and evolve. Every dark moment provides us with the opportunity for high alchemy, the process of taking a very base matter and turning it into gold. If Grace had come into my office for the first time in this moment where she found herself in an overlap, it would immediately signal to me that she is recreating a pattern either from childhood, or familial, cultural, or ancestral trauma, that is asking to be resolved.

Months went by, my condition got worse, and I ended up in hospital. After several painful weeks and medical tests, the doctors told me that I had chronic gastritis and severe irritable bowel syndrome. I had lost so much weight, I could not eat anything. There were days when it took me eight hours to eat a single piece of fruit, as the stomach pain was excruciating. These conditions were a result of the stress I had been enduring for such a long period of time. I knew that this kind of lifestyle was not sustainable long-term. At only 24 years of age, I was on antidepressants, antacids, and by the end of the relationship, I had tried every medication I had heard of to treat my unstable condition.

These digestive symptoms are a classic symptom of Post-Traumatic Stress Disorder. C-PTSD or Complex Post-Traumatic Stress Disorder is defined as complex because it happens consecutively over an extended period of time; for example, recurring childhood physical abuse or sexual abuse has both frequency and longevity. Simple Post-Traumatic Stress Disorder refers to a one-time event, like the loss of a limb from a car accident. In contrast, in recurring traumatic experiences, the body protects and defends itself by going into a survival response—which can range from fight to flight, freeze, or fawn (more on the fawning response later).

When in survival mode, the body responds to danger by shutting down the major organs that require the most blood—stomach, small and large intestines, gall bladder—and sends the blood to the limbs. This makes perfect and logical sense since the rush of blood to the legs and arms prepares the body to run from danger; in danger, eating or drinking are not a priority, escaping the danger is primary.

Over time, however, these fear contractions and responses have a serious impact on the digestive system, especially given that during these cases of abuse or violence, the body is usually immobilized. It's like flooding a car engine with gasoline while it's not moving and doing this over and over. These survival mechanics are showering cortisol throughout the entire system and dramatically shutting down digestion to no avail. This begins to erode and malfunction normal digestive responses. Digestive issues related to PTSD include irritable bowel syndrome, diarrhea, constipation, bloating, stomach ulcers, gall bladder disorders amongst others.

These symptoms are not psychosomatic—they are very real. Because they cannot be correlated to a traditional medical cause, they can seem psychosomatic. I am thankful that in today's emerging medical landscape, the mind-body-spirit connection is being taken very seriously. Please reference Dr. Bessel VanDerKolk, Dr. Gabor Maté, Dr. Judith Orloff, and Dr. Daniel Siegel's work, amongst many others.

After four and a half years of being with this person, I decided that I could not take it anymore, so I built up the courage to end the relationship. It wasn't easy, and having zero friends to support me along the way made everything feel ten times worse, but I wanted to feel happy and alive again. I thought that I had ended my misery, little did I know that the worst was yet to come.

Let's go back to how I met my Prince Charming, who turned out to be my worst nightmare. Just like the typical narcissist, he was extremely attractive, smart, and charismatic, an ambitious journalist by day and a DJ by night.

Only one month had passed since my previous break-up, and I managed to make some new friends who convinced me to start going out partying with them. We met in a nightclub as he was playing music there as a DJ. From the moment I laid eyes on him in the DJ stand, I could not stop thinking about him. There was something different about him; his confidence radiated out of him, and he stood out from everyone. The first time we made eye contact, our eyes locked. I felt it in the very core of my being. I knew that something was going to happen between us, and so it did.

Narcissists are often extremely attractive, intelligent, successful, and charismatic; you can find them in positions of power or experience them as powerful people. Clearly, Grace meeting this person one month after her previous relationship means the pattern was still alive and in full-blown overlap.

Grace's experience of "knowing him" or "knowing something would happen" is not uncommon at all. Sometimes what we feel like a wave of familiarity and amplified attraction is often a familiar pattern, not the person. This attraction is like an echo or a déjà vu, and it is immediately magnetizing. This can be an unconscious memory—deeply buried in the unconscious unless we have worked on it and made it conscious—of someone in our family or in our past who was like this, magnetic, desired, yet dangerous in some way.

The way I like to view this, in a psychospiritual sense, is that we are revisited by the same patterns in order to make new decisions and change our outcomes. I often describe it as it appears, so we can rewrite the end of that chapter in a new way, in our way, in a victorious way, so that we stop feeling powerless in the face of it. We felt and were powerless when the trauma was originally inflicted, and now we can literally change our narrative. Consciousness is the key ingredient to re-creating the story. This all applies to people who are attracted to or co-dependent on people with addictions.

Our relationship started off on the wrong foot from the very beginning. After we noticed each other at the club, we started chatting online. He was very flirty with me, and he started expressing how much he enjoyed speaking with me. We spent hours on end chatting; he was so engaged in the conversation and gave me all kinds of compliments. I could see that he was also smart and intelligent, which I found to be highly attractive qualities. After speaking online and casually meeting for a few weeks, he told me that he had a girlfriend and that he had been in a relationship with her for six years.

The love bombing begins. Love bombing describes the start of a relationship wherein the narcissist, the manipulator, or the groomer (in the case of child abuse) uses extravagant gestures of generosity, affection, praise, attention, even exaggerated kindness, to seduce the other person, who is usually someone who is innocent, naive, lonely, unprotected, wounded, and/or desperate. Characterizing this relational stage as predator and prey is not an exaggeration, mainly because the "predator" knows their end goal, which is to dominate their "prey" for unilateral gain only.

I was devastated as it was too late; I was already under his spell and had already fallen for him hard. I was ashamed of the way I was feeling, and I tried to fight it off because it felt unethical and immoral to get between them. He didn't make it easy for me as he didn't want me to stop speaking to him, and he told me that we should stay in touch as friends and keep it casual. I didn't want to stop meeting him either, guilty as charged. After a few weeks of meeting as friends, we could not resist each other anymore, and we ended up together. Even though I felt extremely guilty because of his girlfriend, I was obsessed with him, yet karma did come back to bite me in the ass.

What Grace is describing here is two ends of the same internal emptiness pole. He begins receiving what is called the "narcissistic supply" from her; in other words, she becomes the gas tank for his need fulfillment and deep sense of inferiority. She overlooks the glaring red flags because of her need for approval, fear of abandonment, or both. They thus begin the dance of co-dependence to fill an emotional need. Our swirling attraction is often the drunken beginnings of codependence.

The energy between us was very intense, we were very passionate with each other, and he seemed like he was as infatuated with me as I was with him. After about one month of juggling between me and his girlfriend, I could not cope with the guilt, and I was super jealous of his girlfriend, whom he spoke very highly of. It did sound a bit strange at the time, and I found myself asking how he could do that to someone he seems to adore and speaks so highly of?

> *It's important to note that Grace's intuition was already speaking, but it gets drowned out by the desperate need to be seen and the fear of abandonment, these are the core Empath wounds. The Empath is a kind of person who not only feels for people, but can actually feel the feelings of others. They are usually highly sensitive, hardworking, and are hard-wired to harmonize environments and keep the peace. They are kind-hearted people who can often play the role of "saviors," "fixers," or "the good child" in their families. Often, they have been overlooked or neglected, so the wounded Empath will have a profound abandonment fear. At the very minimum, the Empath will empathize so deeply with the Narcissist's wound that they find themselves staying longer in an attempt to make them happy, a likely pattern from childhood. The Narcissist will exploit this abandonment wound, and a toxic cycle begins as the Empath becomes the "hard worker" in their relationship in an attempt to "save" the Narcissist and not to be left.*

There were many red flags from the very beginning, the way he was hiding me from his girlfriend was already a sign that he is sneaky and not trustworthy. However, I ignored every sign which indicated that I'm embarking on a very dangerous journey. I insisted, and I made him choose between us because I could not keep sharing him with anyone else. He decided to leave her, and from that day onward, we were inseparable.

After one month of being together, he had asked me to move in with him, and I found this to be quite rushed, but as I mentioned earlier, our relationship was very intense, so I agreed. At the same time, he also informed me that he was still in contact with his ex as they were working together on a project. He reassured me that he was not romantically involved with her, and I believed him. Even though I was not happy with the circumstances, I had no other choice but to accept it, and he informed me that his ex will always be a part of his life. Moving in together didn't happen. He backed down from the plan as he realized that he was rushing, so he told me that we should wait a bit. He still wanted to spend all day and night with me, so I was just happy with that and followed what he said.

As long as he didn't abandon Grace, she'd overlook everything. The red flags thus morphed into self-defeating compromises, boundary busters, and bare minimums.

By the end of the first month, I had many subtle signs that I ignored, especially after throwing a tantrum when he saw me taking a puff from a cigarette at his club for the first time. That night was painful. We went back to his place, and I remember his words loud and clear. He was furious and started telling me that he was disgusted by me, and that he didn't feel attracted to me anymore. I was shocked. How could someone who I thought was so lovely and thoughtful, and who seemed to adore me, turn into this?

He asked me to leave his house and told me that he didn't want to see me anymore. I cried and begged like a dog, and he decided to let me stay with him. The makeup sex was as intense as the argument itself, but back then, I was unaware that I was feeding my egoic need to be validated and desired, rather than making love or fulfilling the need for sexual pleasure.

The core shadow contract was sealed between the two of them: for him, he was now assured that her fear of abandonment anchored her to him so his supply would be endless; for her, she signed her entire self over as his continued presence ratified that she was worth staying for, no matter in what form he stayed, she existed if he stayed.

Just like that, we re-entered the so-called 'love bombing' phase. The initial few months with him felt like pure bliss. He represented everything I was looking for in a guy, and he made me feel like I was the most beautiful girl on the planet. Three months in, and we were already on our first romantic trip. I had planned a surprise birthday holiday to Sicily for him. We were having a fantastic time together until I decided to post our first photo on social media.

He threw a raging tantrum and turned into this cold-hearted person whom I could not recognize. I felt like he was ashamed of me and that he wanted to hide me away from someone. This experience describes our entire relationship, alternating between an amazing period of time (love bombing phase) and dismissal time.

Narcissistic punishments follow a well-trodden trajectory, whether it be from a parent, boss, or lover, and it includes the silent treatment, affection withdrawal, berating, gaslighting, aggression, and even violence. Grace's depiction of this cyclical push and pull as a drug craving is right on the money. This power play, which is at the very center of the Narcissist/

Empath relationship, is a relational addiction. Like an addiction, there is a constant "chasing the high" to fulfill a profound, existential emptiness. Notice that they both have it, just at the opposite ends of the spectrum.

Narcissists have a way of withdrawing their love and affection from you, and the way they manage to hook you on them, you end up craving them like a drug. Back then, I had no idea what was going on; I had never even heard the term narcissistic personality disorder, let alone what it meant.

We both really enjoyed traveling, and after eight months of dating, we decided to go on another trip as he got invited to a family wedding in South America, and he asked me to join him. I was super excited because this was my first trip out of Europe, and it seemed like my traveling dreams were finally coming true.

We had already broken up twice until it was time to go on this holiday, as he was feeling uncertain about us. To my surprise, what I imagined to be an exciting and romantic trip to South America turned out to be a big disappointment with a lot of heartache. For the first time ever, I started to see his personality coming out. I noticed that he really enjoyed speaking about himself and that he wasn't much interested in listening to what other people had to say. He bragged for hours on end about his personal successes, and he seemed really inconsiderate when it came to other people's feelings.

To the narcissist, the other person—including their own children—is just an object. No one else truly exists, and everyone is measured according to their capacity to "supply," in this case, as a receptacle of his ravings, monologues, or as a trophy. There is no dyad or other person. The relationship is emotionally masturbatory.

It was New Year's Eve, and we spent the night overlooking the mountains in Chile with his family. The view was spectacular, it seemed like the perfect way to spend New Year's Eve, yet I felt completely alone, as if I were invisible. This practically describes how I felt throughout our relationship, as he never paid attention to me in social gatherings. He liked showing me around as his girlfriend, as if I were some kind of trophy, but that was just about it.

When I tried to speak in social gatherings, he used to put me down and shut me up. Later on, he informed me that I was not allowed to speak in public because I was boring and not up to his standard. We had countless fights, which got more heated as time went by, and I wasn't one to hold back when it came to calling him out on his lies.

By the end of the relationship, I could not take the lies anymore, and at that point, I found it difficult to tell what was real or not. Early in the relationship, he had already lost my trust, as it wasn't the first time that I saw him chatting and flirting with other girls. When I confronted him, he was always ready to defend himself and make up excuses to justify his behavior. For some reason, even though I didn't believe him, I still decided to continue seeing him. Since he switched from being fun and affectionate, to a cold-hearted liar, I always kept hoping that things would change for the better. So, I just held on to the good moments.

Like an addiction, we unconsciously are addicted to the hope that "this time it will be different," and it never is. Like Grace, the Empath wonders, "Maybe this time the chapter will end differently," so the Empath stays and stays. This hope that the story will end differently (very likely the childhood wounded story that the current relationship is emulating and attempting to heal), becomes a destructive, repetitive glitch when it doesn't correct or up-level the original relational trauma.

Intermittent "highs" are the characteristic of most addictions, and we keep wanting to get back to the original high. The narcissist is so delicious during the love bombing stage and seems to have the capacity to see the Empath so fully, and this is actually genuine. The narcissist is seeing the Empath in great, elaborate detail because they are assessing the level of supply the Empath's desperate need to be seen will provide. Can you see how the narcissist and the wounded Empath are a perfect match? It is like a plug into a socket. The narcissist is exquisitely attuned at the beginning, but only because they are detailing their prey and the likelihood of being able to dominate them completely. A more healed Empath will not do because their boundary markings would be more pronounced and would completely repel the true Narcissist. Basically, they are reading the Empath quite specifically, which makes the Empath feel known and adored.

This attunement never returns and is replaced by its opposite, a constant "unseeing," which is why Grace feels so invisible. This is the original trauma "glitch" that not only never heals in this type of relationship, it exacerbates.

After about three years together, I was finally able to understand the reason behind his erratic behavior and why I was going through such a confusing and painful time. I was talking to one of my girlfriends, and I was sharing my pain and distress with her. She had been a witness to our relationship, which felt like an emotional roller coaster, and one day she said it out loud and told me that he sounds narcissistic.

I had never heard of this term before, and I started doing some research about it. Everything made sense, the lies, the manipulation, the tantrums, the lack of empathy, getting blamed for everything, the list goes on. The description of what it meant to be with someone who had a narcissistic personality disorder perfectly described what I was going through. I had empathized with him and felt a great sense of compassion for him because I understood that this issue came from his unresolved emotional childhood trauma.

> *This is a dangerous place for the Empath who is gifted with seeing someone else's point of view and feeling the other's wound. This can keep the Empath in the relationship for a long time--and the Narcissist will milk it. The guilt of abandoning the narcissist, the Empath's very own worst fear, traps them in the relationship. I have coined this "emotional molestation."*
>
> *Emotional molestation is when the predatory authority figure, parent, or partner intentionally molests the child's or Empath's kind heart through fear, guilt, or shame. Emotional molestation is as erosive as sexual molestation in that it abuses the kind heart as it does the body in sexual molestation. Boundaries are invaded, and souls are crushed in the process with long-term traumatic ramifications.*

I had many debates with myself to see how I was going to speak to him about it and see his reaction. One day, I built up the courage and wrote him a letter. The letter was full of warm words of unconditional love and acceptance of the situation. I gave it to him and let him read it, and his reaction left me speechless.

He didn't look surprised at all. He told me that he knew about it and that he never really felt the need to mention it. I was shocked, and I asked him how long he had known and when he had figured it out. He told me that when he was studying for his bachelor's degree in psychology, he recognized these behavioral traits and patterns within himself. He even said that, if anything, this made him more special and superior to others because, in his eyes, other people were just basic. I was shocked by this response. That was the moment I slowly started to realize just how serious this problem actually was. But he played it very cool when

I confronted him, as if he wasn't bothered at all by the conversation. However, he couldn't look me in the eye after that.

My presence reminded him of who he was, and it was too uncomfortable for him to face it. As you can imagine, the fights were happening on a daily basis, and every day he reminded me of how useless I was. He used to invent things to blame me for and go on for hours belittling me and telling me that I had no skills whatsoever. After hearing the same thing over and over again, you start to believe it yourself. You completely lose touch with who you are, and your mind feels foggy and confused all the time. All you can think about is how to make things better, to get you both out of that misery.

I call this the "glazing over" and the "narcissistic haze." It's important to recognize them both as signals in future moments of identifying red flags. What happens is that the Empath's (or others') central nervous system has been pummeled, their reality questioned so consistently, and their need to keep the peace vis-à-vis the constant conflict creates a zombie-like demeanor.

Remember, the Empath or most humans, will want to harmonize an environment, and when in a relationship with a narcissist, this human, organic function goes into overdrive. Since there is no winning and no mutuality with the narcissist, the Empath, the child, or the other, moves into a "narcissistic haze" and "glazes over." In clinical language, we call it disassociation, which is a defensive measure, a checking out, in the face of danger and trauma. They literally must leave their bodies in order to survive their environment.

Over time, this defensive mechanism, disassociation, can become a way of being in the world. Over a long period of time, and if in constant contact with the narcissist, the person fully "glazes over," gets sick, and even dies because their being has been completely decimated. Either way, it is a psychic or physical death. These words are not an over-dramatization; I have worked with and studied case after case of this predictable prognosis.

The Empath is hard wired to harmonize environments. So the work is endless and empty with the NPD because the environment is never harmonized. Mindfully noticing your moments of feeling "hazy" or "glazed over" around people or situations is important so that you can discern if you're in the presence of a narcissist or having a defensive response for whatever reason. Mindfulness and spiritual self-attunement are essential practices in the recovery process in order to notice dissociative moments, which could be signaling a red flag or an overwhelming experience. A trauma-informed therapist will also help notice moments of disassociation.

Being the codependent person that I was back then, I felt responsible for the situation, and I made it my problem to fix. So, I suggested that we move in together as a trial. I was sure that my love for him one day would be enough to resolve the issue. I wanted to make things work against all odds, ignoring all the flirting and lies and the stress my body was going through. With a sense of trepidation, we decided to move in together to try it out for a couple of months. We entered the apartment arguing, and we spent our very first night there sleeping in separate bedrooms. Six months later, when the rental agreement came to an end, we left the apartment screaming at each other and went our separate ways.

Living with him was very intense and stressful. He rarely helped out with cleaning or cooking and was always finding things to complain about. Cooking for him was not an easy task, and sometimes after hours of cooking for him, he used to throw big fights and punish me for using the wrong ingredient. I lost count of how many times I had to move out of our main bedroom and sleep in the spare bedroom for a whole weekend and get the silent treatment.

He played a lot of mind games with me to demonstrate his power and control over me, and I could see him enjoying it in his eyes each time he succeeded. Whatever happened, he never took the blame or apologized, and everything had to happen according to his terms. I started feeling like I was trapped with him. He used to get very irritated if he didn't find me at home at certain times. Not being there to attend to his needs left him feeling frustrated. It wasn't the first time that he said out loud that he felt entitled to receiving special treatment and using someone for his own benefit, and I could feel that I was one of his victims. At the same time, I couldn't imagine being without him.

Grace's experience of being unable to leave him, despite being aware that the situation was worsening, is known as "learned helplessness." Learned helplessness is a term used for people trapped in an abusive cycle wherein, after being psychologically and often physically abused over a long period of time, they can no longer see solutions or options, even when they are there. The key component here is not being able to see a viable exit, even when it exists.

This is an actual psychological phenomenon that occurs with abused children, prisoners of war, and domestic abuse cases. Knowing about learned helplessness is essential for having compassion for these victims who are often judged and misunderstood for not leaving or escaping; yet the learned helplessness cognitive distortion and its accompanying terror have enlarged to a degree that blinds the individual to possibilities. Psycho-spiritually speaking, the belief that possibility is non-existent is the ultimate enslavement of the human, and it is how trauma robs us of the experience of planning a future.

We had broken up many times, but we always ended up together after just a couple of days. After about three months living together, it was time for another holiday. There wasn't one single holiday where it didn't involve me crying and fighting, but this holiday was a before-and-after kind of holiday.

I had booked a place in Budapest, and we decided to go there for an event during my birthday week. The event happened to be on the first night, so we hit the ruin bars and went to the event. It was all good until we started fighting in the venue. The argument escalated quickly, and I ended up chasing him as he started running away from me. It was around 04.00 am and I was drunk by that time. I didn't want to be left alone as I wasn't feeling capable of taking care of myself. At some point, he pushed me into the crowd, and a security guy happened to see him. The security guard grabbed him and threw him out of the club.

This type of emotional sadism is the mark of an individual with full-blown NPD. At this point in the relationship, there was no more hiding his actual intentions for using Grace as a supply source because he had tested her enough, and she had stayed through almost all his boundary violations. Grace here is stuck in a downward spiral of intense fear of abandonment, of rapidly decreasing self-esteem, and of feeling less and less worthy of healed love, thus multiplying her abandonment fear. Some internal questions that happen at this point are, "Who else would love me?" "Who would want me like this?" "Who am I without this person?" The sense of self is slowly eroding, and the thought of going out into the rest of the world alone is experienced as more dangerous than staying with the abusive narcissist. This is what is called cognitive distortion. Cognitive distortions are mental schemas or models that exacerbate suffering, are the main contributors to anxiety and depression, and make us feel bad about ourselves.

It's important to note that Grace running after him when he walks away is an automatic response from her inner child. Walking away is a punishing behavior and exploits her fear of abandonment, and likely, what Grace was not able to do as a child—run after a caregiver or plead for love—she automatically and unconsciously does as an adult. The alcohol puts her in a semi-conscious state, and so her primal instincts are more impulsive. This is her inner child pleading to not be left. Again, for the reader or the victim, understanding these behaviors that may seem desperate or illogical from an outsider perspective provides a framework of compassion within which to put them. These are profound wounds that resurface, and the opportunity here is to see them for what they are and offer them healing.

I knew that I would be punished and held responsible for his humiliation. I followed him out of the venue, and he started shouting at me, and he left running to our apartment. I didn't know the address where we were staying, so I panicked and started running after him. It was January in Budapest, so the floor was covered with thin ice, and chasing your boyfriend while drunk is not the best idea. As I was running, I slipped on the ice and smashed my face and body on the floor. I stood up and saw him running. I looked down and I noticed that my face was covered in blood. My whole body was aching, and when I looked around, I saw an ambulance and asked for help.

From a holistic perspective—mind, body, and spirit—our internal wounds will begin to appear in our external world if we don't heed their call. Accidents, sickness, physical pain, and disease are signs that a psychological wound is festering. Our spirit, through our body, will try to get our attention at increasing rates in an attempt to have us self-heal and self-love. If something is happening in or on your body, ask, "How might this be connected to my internal state?"

Can you see here that Grace's desperate need for attention and validation was getting louder and more dramatic? The security guard noticed and protected her; the ambulance people helped her and cared for her. Her inner child is begging to be cared for and is asking in louder ways. All of this is unconscious which is why it is helpful to ask, "What is my body trying to tell me?"

To make things worse, the medical staff did not speak English, but they cleaned my face, and they were trying to understand what had happened to me. Suddenly, I saw him a bit distant from the ambulance, and I left to go meet him. I was limping and my mouth was destroyed as I chipped a tooth and broke my braces. We started walking home and continued fighting. I remember walking in the middle of the streets, crying and hoping that a car would hit me to end the pain.

Grace's desperation begins to form into "passive suicidality." Passive suicidality is a desire to die without having an actual plan and with fantasies that it happens inadvertently, like getting hit by a car or slipping and falling.

Instead of asking me to go over to him or try to protect me in any way, he took out his mobile phone and started taking a video and making fun of me. Cars were stopping and shouting at me. I don't blame them. I had completely lost my mind, and I wanted my nightmare to end.

Somehow, we made it back home, and he went on for hours telling me how much he hated me and that I ruined his life. Not once had he asked me how I felt or if I needed anything. After hours of crying and listening to his venomous words, we fell asleep. The next morning, I looked in the mirror and I was horrified, I had never seen myself that way.

My face was bruised, my lips were swollen, I chipped my tooth, broke my braces, and had two large bruises on my chest and thighs. I called my orthodontist, and he told me that I need to get them fixed as soon as possible. I panicked, and I didn't know what to do at the time. I called my sister and my friends to seek support, but I was terrified at the same time because he was always telling me to keep things private. They advised me to seek medical assistance over there, so when he woke up, I planned to try to convince him to take me to a clinic.

When he woke up, he insisted on getting sexual favors and immediately started belittling me and telling me how useless I was. Another fight started, and after four hours of agony listening to him, he left the apartment and went sightseeing. I stayed crying alone, waiting for him to come back, feeling completely helpless. He came back after a while and asked me to go to a spa the next day. I agreed, and we spent one hour walking to the spa because he felt like walking despite the fact that I was limping all the way through.

At this point, Grace is a severely wounded and abused Empath and is fully experiencing learned helplessness. She has the guidance to seek help, has the available exit to get care while he is gone, and yet does not take the opportunity. Furthermore, the desperate Empath or victim will be grateful for any crumbs, so his suggestion to go to the spa together, which seems like a non-abandoning gesture, feels like care. It is worth noting that it is actually the NPD who needs Grace, as he keeps coming back in spite of "hating her" and claiming that she is "ruining his life." He also has the opportunity to leave at any moment—and anyone who is more healed might truly leave this peak abusive moment—but neither does. This is a putrefying, co-dependent and co-created cycle.

He started taking photos of my bruised face and laughing at me, remarking at how ugly I looked with a grin on his face. By the time we arrived at the spa, I couldn't feel my leg anymore, and I wanted to get it checked out. As soon as I expressed my need to go to a clinic, he started shouting at me and telling me that I was ruining his day and messing up his itinerary. He gave me an ultimatum and told me that the only way he was taking me to a clinic was if I booked a flight and left the next day.

Grace, by requesting help and putting her needs first, thus informs him that she is becoming a decreasing source for his supply, and so he asks her to leave. Any sign of supply depletion will not be tolerated.

I was desperate at that point and for the first time ever, it sounded relieving to get away from him. So I agreed, and we went to the closest hospital. While we were waiting, he tormented me for hours, and I just couldn't wait to get away from him. I booked a flight while waiting at the hospital, and I left the following day.

Returning home without him was still painful, and when my friends and family saw the state I was in, they were shocked. From that day onward, they never spoke to him again, and I defended him as always. I went back to our place, trying to figure out how to survive the next few days while he was still enjoying himself in Budapest. I looked in the mirror and I noticed that my face looked dull and lifeless.

I call this the "zombie" look, which is beyond being "glazed over" or disassociated; literally, the NPD codependent becomes the "walking dead."

No words can describe the amount of pain I was feeling; my heart was completely broken, along with my identity and self-esteem. Suddenly a thought popped up and I remembered that his laptop was in our bedroom, so I went to have a look at it. I was not proud of what I was about to do, but I couldn't hold back considering the circumstances, and my gut feeling was telling me that he's up to something. By then, I could predict his behavior, and the more I learned about narcissistic personality disorder, the easier it became for me to predict him. He followed it like a script, so I was always one step ahead of him. When I opened his laptop, I saw that he was already on Tinder, planning his first date. He had booked a romantic dinner for me for my birthday on the Danube River in Budapest.

Knowing him, he wasn't going to waste such a good opportunity to sweep a girl off her feet. So, he replaced me with a girl he had matched with on Tinder and took her to my birthday dinner date. He took her back to the place we were staying (which *I* had paid for). I was furious. How could he?! I was sure that I'd had enough and decided to end the relationship with him as soon as he came back.

The following days were extremely painful, as soon as I opened my eyes in the morning, I used to feel a rush of panic taking over my whole body, and my heart used to start racing. I could not focus on anything, and his words were stuck in my head, repeating over and over again how useless and stupid I was. I started asking myself what had happened to the amazing, charming, and intelligent person I had fallen in love with? It seemed like he never really existed!

These are C-PTSD symptoms that are emerging as they do, even if we are away from the actual danger. The mind, body, and spirit have now memorized the terror. Notice here that Grace is still wondering about where he went, and yet the important spiritual question is, where did beautiful, intelligent, and vibrant Grace go?

The following morning, I decided to go have breakfast by myself for the first time. It felt a bit weird, but I built up some courage and ordered a lovely meal by the sea. I still remember how beautiful it was eating in perfect silence. For once, I was eating in peace, without having to listen to him rambling for hours and transmitting his negative energy to me. I truly appreciated and enjoyed that moment; it was a milestone in my transformation, as it was my first act of self-love, taking myself out on a date for a tasty breakfast.

Unfortunately, soon after my peace was broken, when he came back, we went for brunch as if nothing had happened, and he turned on his charm. Within a few minutes, I was already swept off my feet, and he managed to manipulate me to accept what had happened. I confronted him about his romance in Budapest, and he denied it at first. When I showed him that I had proof, he immediately started to play the victim and defend himself to justify his behavior. Even though it did not make sense to me, I let him push my boundaries once again, and I accepted him back. My friends and family were furious when I told them that we were back together, and looking back, I can see why.

The isolating shame begins, and friends and family don't understand the depth and gravity of Grace's desperation to "finally" change his narrative of her. At this point, it's not only his NPD abuse that is the problem; it's Grace's locked-in codependency.

The relationship didn't get easier, and we were fighting on a daily basis. He told me that in five years, I hadn't earned his respect because I hadn't proven to him that I had any skills or that I was worthy of anything. It was very confusing, as there were other days when he counterargued these statements, telling me how much he loved me and how special I was to him.

We had many discussions about his behavior and how the personality disorder was affecting our relationship, but I never got anywhere with him. The following day he used to deny having those discussions and he used to twist whatever we had agreed upon during the conversation. I started recording our conversations so the next time he denied saying something, I thought bringing out the evidence would show him how much he was lying.

This plan backfired, as when I showed him our conversation, he would get furious and accuse me of being crazy.

This is classic gaslighting. Gaslighting is an intentional and strategic manipulation to have the other—the victim or the abused Empath—question their sense of reality, their perceptions, or their memory of an event. Grace's inner self is telling her to record the conversations so that she can prove to him—and to herself!—that what she heard or saw was real. Calling her crazy is a gaslighting technique and can also make the victim feel "crazy" because the act of recording a conversation as proof does feel out of the norm for themselves. The victim feels like their behavior is erratic, and it merges with his description of her.

He was scared and worried that I was recording him to use the recordings as evidence in court, but I assured him that I had no intention of escalating things.

Back then I believed him, but now that I know what kind of tactics these people use, I know that he was just diverting the point of the argument to avoid what I originally wanted to say to him. I could never win with him no matter what I did, and I was feeling mentally exhausted as if someone was sucking out all my energy. We couldn't take it anymore, so we decided to break up and stay living under the same roof as friends. As you can imagine, this wasn't easy for me, but for him, this was the best case scenario, and he managed to get exactly what he wanted.

He had always been telling me that he had an open relationship with his ex-girlfriend, and even though he did not want to share me with anyone, the same rules didn't apply to him. So, this way he was free to flirt and see other girls, while having me at the same time whenever he felt like it. I wasn't happy about this, but I had become so submissive at that point that he could do anything with me, and I just followed along. We kept this agreement until the end of the contract, and when it was time to leave the apartment, we left screaming at each other. Our neighbors must have been happy to see us leave. I wasn't in good shape, I was extremely stressed and anxious, and I couldn't find peace no matter what I did.

This is a trauma response called hypervigilance. It is a chronic state of feeling like something dangerous will happen. Hypervigilance gets memorized in the body and it occurs after being in an actual war, after being violated or abused, and if growing up in a chaotic, disorganized home, amongst others. The internal state feels electrical, hyper alert, and suspicious. When I am teaching emotional regulation, I like to identify this internal state as code yellow, code orange, or code red, as a way of measuring the sense of dread and thus assist in calibrating it. What is notable about hypervigilance is that it is now inside the body, whether there is an external danger or not.

My sister recommended a healer to help me process what I was going through, and I am truly grateful for taking this step, as it was the beginning of my transformation. When I started seeing my healer, I used to burst out crying before I had even started speaking. I was so overwhelmed with all the pain and emotions, I felt like I had completely lost touch with myself. The healer used to teach me techniques on how to process all the emotions and release them, but this was a slow process, and I understood that it takes time to heal.

I realized that I had a lot of work to do, but I wanted to work on myself and understand why this had happened to me and why I allowed someone to take advantage of me. For some reason, I stayed in a toxic relationship, and during my sessions, it became clear that I had a codependency issue. Practicing meditation helped me to get more clarity on these kinds of issues as I started to enhance my self-awareness and understand myself better.

Introspection sheds light on your shadows, and I had to face my biggest fears if I wanted to strengthen myself and heal. The more I worked on myself, the more I started to feel empowered, and I started seeing some improvement in my life. Unfortunately, it wasn't long until he sucked me back into his toxicity.

Narcissists make it hard for you to leave, and at that time, I thought it was because he loved me. But now I understand that narcissistic people do this not because they love you, but because they want to keep taking advantage of you and prove to themselves that they still have power over you. I fell for his charm once again, and we ended up back together. My friends and family didn't accept this, and since he never really spent time with them, this wasn't really a problem. I had told him that I was seeing a healer, and he wasn't happy to hear this, as he knew that this was a threat to his power over me.

Grace's points are accurate, and I would add another factor that is more disguised and hard to see in the narcissist because of their grandiosity: the narcissist has an extreme sense of internal emptiness and loneliness that can NEVER be filled, which is why they seek constant sources of emotional supply. As I always say, spoiler alert: it's the narcissist that never leaves (even though they consistently threaten to leave, as a tactic for keeping their supplier on pins and needles).

This is an emotional molestation of the Empath's or victims abandonment/neglect wound; yet it's the narcissist who has extreme fears of being abandoned. They project their "not enoughness" onto the supplier—"you're not enough and never will be, which is why I need to seek other people"—and appear like a cheater or a player, and yet, at its core, all it is a desperate attempt to not be left alone.

To make me feel ashamed for seeking support, he started calling me crazy and that my healer was even crazier than me. He wanted me to stay weak and vulnerable so he could easily manipulate me. I couldn't bear staying with him anymore, and I decided to end it. By the end of the relationship, the passion had dissolved, he never wanted to do anything fun with me, and I just had to sit there listening to him talking about his work and successes for hours. The relationship was always one-sided; he never really nurtured me or took care of my needs. Women kept getting between us, he was like a magnet to them. I'm not surprised. He was very charismatic and charming, and he knew exactly what to say to make someone fall for him.

Everyone liked him in the beginning; he is a very interesting and talented person, but if you get close enough, it's only a matter of time until reality hits you.

This is another example of the mirage; it's quite mesmerizing, seductive, and extremely difficult to see past it, especially if you yourself are in need of validation. This type of attention feels like the lottery.

By the end of the relationship, I felt like I was wasting my time with him and that I could never be happy in the future living like this. I still continued working on myself during the last few months of being with him, and I'm sure that it played a major role in finally opening up my eyes and seeing him for who he really was. A few months after starting the sessions, I decided to set myself free as I realized that I could have a much better life without him. I got in touch with my inner power and started practicing self-love and self-compassion. Change was uncomfortable at first, but I was feeling much better, so I opened myself up to new possibilities and made peace with what had happened to me.

One of the major reasons that made it difficult for me to leave the narcissist was that I felt like I never had closure. We broke up and got back together countless times because every time I thought I would confront him to get some closure, he always managed to manipulate the conversation and make me fall for his charm. It was difficult for me to move on because he never admitted that he had done anything wrong, so he never apologized for the pain he caused me.

Grace's point here about closure is so important for the healing to begin! It is, in fact, the key. The addictive cycle is centered around craving a different narrative, a different ending to the story, and yet it's you—or in this case, Grace—who has to provide this ending, not the narcissist. Spiritually, we see these as cycles of learning, some circles would call this karma. The situation will appear over and over again until we re-write how it ends or shifts or evolves. The redesign is in our hands, not anyone else's.

Once I made peace with the fact that he can never give me closure, it was a kind of closure in itself as I had accepted the situation. I accepted the fact that he was behaving with me the way he was, not because I was doing something wrong or because I wasn't good enough, but because of his mental health issues. The more I learned about narcissism and about myself, the more I could understand what had happened and learned from it.

For the first time in my life, I started doing things that felt good to me and stopped trying to please everyone around me. If you are a codependent, you know exactly what I'm talking about, as you always find yourself going out of your way to help others. The more I practiced meditation, the more I was able to bring these fragments into my conscious mind, and I could work on them to change my behavior and make better choices for my life and emotional well-being.

This is the blissful return to SELF! The coming home to whom we are. Tara Brach, a psycho-spiritual teacher like myself, says that "all sickness is homesickness." We are away from our most treasured home: the self.

I cannot express enough gratitude for my healer, who was a catalyst in my transformation. He had helped me liberate myself from my abuser, and most importantly from my self-limitations. When I started working on myself, it was the first time that I showed up for myself and was determined to stay committed to set myself free. I embarked on an exciting journey of self-discovery, and I was finally able to be happy with myself without seeking external validation and approval from others. Going no contact with my ex was the best choice I could have made as I eliminated every chance of falling for his manipulative lies again.

When it comes to an individual with narcissistic personality disorder—whether it be a lover, family member, friend, or boss—going no contact is the only answer. These are not people who are likely to work on themselves, even when they say they will, and once you leave they will promise you everything! That is why it takes several rounds before leaving them.

No contact seems very dramatic and final, because it is. This is non-negotiable. If you're an Empath, there is more to discuss about this because it will seem very drastic and unkind, and feeling unkind goes against their very core nature, but sadly contributes to the entrapment. In my book, The Empath Leader, I explore in depth ways to commit to the kind heart, while also maintaining boundaries of self-love and self-respect. More on this later.

When I ended the relationship, it was still painful and heavy, it felt like my life had ended with a strong sense of emptiness and lack of purpose. Little did I know that it was just the beginning of the most liberating and beautiful experience on this planet, waking up to who I really am and the ultimate reality.

Part II

The Psychology Behind NPD & Narcissistic Abuse

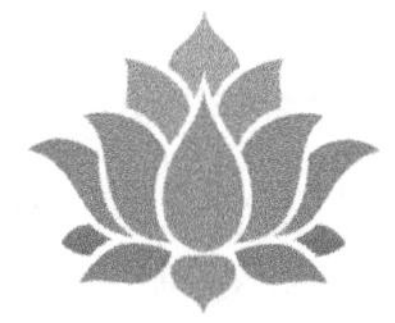

UNDERSTANDING HOW NARCISSISTS WORK was the first step towards my healing process. In this section, I would like to give you some information about Narcissistic Personality Disorder (NPD). It will help you realize that what happened is not your fault. Even though you might feel that you are not good enough, or that you keep messing things up, this is just what the narcissist wants you to believe.

Learning about the psychology behind narcissistic personality disorder really helped me understand what I was going through. Prior to learning about it, I spent all my days fixated on our relationship, trying to make sense out of things, and failed miserably. When I started to learn about it, I realized that no matter how hard I tried, I was not going to fix the issue. I spent weeks reading and learning about it, and I started following online support groups for victims of narcissistic abuse. These groups helped me feel understood and comforted as I realized that I was not alone, and all of us were going through similar situations. All the victims in the support group were describing their situations, and we could see that we were all experiencing the same things in a different setting or context.

What Grace did here is transmute a negative experience, energy, or focus—in this case, obsessive ruminations about her partner and the relationship—by funneling it into her self-knowledge and self-healing. These are specific signs of the start of the healing journey, when we redirect all the energy we gave towards our addictive patterns towards our well-being. We can call this a fuel source. Some good questions are what is my fuel source, and where am I putting it?

Learning about NPD is just the beginning of the healing process. You start healing and seeing effective changes in your life when you shift your focus to your relationship with yourself. By asking yourself the right questions, you begin to understand yourself on a deeper level. Self-awareness and introspection shed light on why you chose to stick around with a person who made your life miserable. Only then can you set yourself free from the unresolved emotional wounds that got you into the toxic relationship in the first place.

Chapter 2

NPD: Causes & Indicative Signs

I WILL NEVER FORGET HOW he smirked in triumph when he looked at my bruised face following my accident in Budapest. My perception of him changed that day. When I looked into his eyes, I saw a heartless monster, and I couldn't wrap my head around the fact that he was laughing out loud and pointing out how ugly I looked. How could someone behave like that? You don't even treat strangers like that, let alone someone you claim to love. I remember asking myself, *'Am I dealing with a psychopath?'*

> *This is what I call the "why" chapter of the relationship, and it can be an extremely long chapter in life. Whether it be an abusive parent, the school bully, the constantly critical boss, or the heartless partner, we ask ourselves "why" for a very long time. "I'm your daughter, Why do you hate me so much?" "I'm doing everything you asked, why isn't it enough?" "I'm keeping to myself, why do you come after me to humiliate me?" The abusive bully shows up in dictators and in systems as well. "I was born into this religion, or I was born into this race, why would you annihilate me for this?"*

We truly don't understand why someone can be so cruel, and this is a high, logical, human question because we are organically born with an ability to care. The challenge is that while we are in an abusive relationship or situation, we can get stuck asking why, and it becomes a very circular place, leading to obsessions, ruminations, and chronic hoop-jumping to change it while all the while it becomes worse.

The scientific evidence behind NPD helped me understand how a human being is able to be so cruel and malicious. According to a study conducted by researchers at PsychCentral, narcissists have been found to exhibit less gray matter, which may be associated with their lack of empathy ("Narcissists' Lack of Empathy," 2013). Personality disorders are developed over time as a result of certain genetic components and childhood experiences. It is common that kids and adolescents have some narcissistic traits and seem self-centered, but this does not mean that each and every one of them will develop a full-blown disorder.

Narcissistic personality disorder continues to develop throughout the teenage years or young adulthood and can result from several different scenarios and experiences. The following circumstances, combined with genetic factors, can lead to developing NPD: being excessively praised for good behaviors or excessively criticized for bad behaviors; learning manipulative behaviors from parents; suffering from childhood abuse or neglect; inconsistent parental caregiving; being excessively admired and receiving excessive praise focused on your looks or skills. These factors play an important role in an individual's self-esteem, especially later on in adolescence.

Narcissists might seem to have an inflated, high self-esteem, but at the same time, they are super fragile and depend on external validation to feel good about themselves. They believe grandiose fantasies about themselves either about their physical appearance or intellectual abilities, and they easily put other people down to make themselves feel superior. Individuals with NPD tend to exaggerate their accomplishments and successes, and they feel entitled to exploit other people for personal gain. They manipulate others by gaslighting people, and as a result, their victims end up questioning their own thoughts, memories, and the events occurring around them.

Victims of gaslighting end up questioning their own sanity as they start questioning their own reality due to the emotional manipulation and the constant lies they are faced with. Another manipulation technique that they use is arguing about a particular event and redefining reality with fictional details as if they were facts. They can be extremely convincing, and their victims end up questioning whether narcissists believe their own lies. Eventually, this kind of redefining reality leads victims to question their own understanding of reality and to end up feeling high levels of anxiety and depression.

This is what I call emotional molestation, a phrase I have coined with specific reference to narcissism. Emotional molestation is when someone with a kind heart, like a child, an Empath, or anyone who is willing to see the good in people and believes in care and reciprocity, is manipulated with the use of guilt, shame, or fear. There is a spectrum of emotional molestation: gaslighting, humiliation, verbal, sexual, and physical abuse are on the most toxic polarity.

When I had learned all of this, everything made sense. No wonder I was recording our conversations. I used to repeatedly listen to our conversations because of his continuous tweaking of facts and events. Gaslighting is extremely damaging as it destroys your ability to trust yourself. My sense of intuition and perception of reality were completely demolished. I felt paralyzed without any sense of direction. Our intuition acts as an internal compass, an internal guidance system that guides us in our life journey. But how can you know which direction to take if your internal compass is broken?

This moment is classic in terms of the swirly self-doubt that begins to happen, including feeling confused and having to record. Even though Grace describes feeling that her internal compass was broken—and yes, this was happening and happens!—Her intuition was trying to stay alive by saying, "Record this. You're right. Chart evidence that supports you." Spiritually speaking, her inner being was fighting. I believe so much in tracking the times our inner being was showing up for us because those are times when our Higher Self is providing us signals out of the darkness.

I was at his mercy, powerless and easily manipulated. At this point, I didn't trust my emotions, my thoughts, or my perceptions. He shaped my reality with his discourse, and he implanted beliefs in my head about myself and about the world that were extremely harmful and completely false. But at the time, I believed them, so they were very real to me. Losing the ability to trust myself was the biggest hurdle that I had to overcome.

Through meditation and spirituality, I was able to reclaim myself and strengthen my sense of intuition. Strengthening your intuition helps you become self-reliant and feel supported and guided along your journey.

This is so powerful. I am reminded of the biblical story of Samson's hair being cut or Superman being weakened by kryptonite. Losing trust in ourselves is when humans can be completely enslaved. Knowing and trusting oneself is a human superpower. It makes logical sense that it's what the narcissist tries to disassemble first.

Let's recap the main symptoms of narcissistic personality disorder according to Mayo Clinic ("Narcissistic Personality Disorder," n.d.):

- Grandiose sense of self
- Exaggerated fantasies of success, power, glory, beauty, or ideal love
- Perceive themselves as special, unique, and above standard. They believe that they should only associate with other special or high-status people or organizations
- Need for excessive and constant admiration
- Feel entitled to special treatment
- Exploitative behavior with others
- Lack of empathy
- Envy of others or imagining that others are envious of them
- Arrogant and disdainful behaviors or attitudes

As you can see, these qualities make it very difficult to build a healthy and loving relationship where both parties have equal power in the relationship. Choosing to stay with a person who possesses these traits means that you are condemning yourself to a lifetime of suffering, neglect, and different forms of abuse. Why would anyone want to sign up for that kind of future?

Even though it sounds crazy to stay in this kind of relationship, many of us do, and I was one of them. To understand why you have made this choice, or why you are still choosing this kind of relationship, you need to dig deeper to see what kind of beliefs and ideas you have about yourself and the world around you.

INSIGHTFUL LESSON: What the narcissist tells you about yourself and the world is not true. Be brave and find your truth. It *will* set you free.

Releasing the Pain

Step 1: Close your eyes and take three deep, mindful breaths.

Step 2: Put one hand on your heart and one hand on your stomach. Take a moment to be with yourself and observe the rhythm of your breath flow.

Step 3: Let your emotions surface so you can release them out of your body. If you feel the need to cry, let it all out. Crying is a way of releasing pain; otherwise, it will stay trapped in your body, which can be detrimental to your physical health.

Step 4: Wrap your hands around yourself and give yourself a hug. Repeat this statement to yourself and return to this statement whenever the need arises: *"I love myself, and I promise myself that I will protect myself. I know deep within my heart that what the narcissist tells me about myself is not true. I let go of negative beliefs about myself. From now onwards, I give myself permission to connect with who I really am and to find my truth."*

Take three more mindful breaths. What does your heart tell you about the relationship?

If you feel that you need to seek support and speak with a therapist to help you manage your emotions, it can help a great deal in the process of healing. I know that this process might be painful, but trust me, there's a whole new beautiful world on the other side of healing, waiting for you to find it. When you start going within yourself, you will realize that you are beyond what you ever imagined.

The Dynamic Meditation Method (Dynamic for short) is an amalgam of concepts, tools, and processes that I created to expedite and anchor my psychotherapy clients' healing. I use Dynamic for emotional regulation and self-mastery. Grace has requested that in the exercise section of this book, I add some of these Dynamic exercises.

It may be helpful to know that I myself am a trauma survivor and have experienced extremely intense configurations of that trauma, which included high anxiety, panic attacks, a 10-year phobia, severe abandonment fear, and hypervigilance. I used the Dynamic Meditation Method on myself first, and it entirely healed me. I found that I had to create something for people like me who could be—at first—triggered by sitting still and quietly, because the mind is still an internalized abuser and the body is saturated with electrical short-circuits. Hence, please know that these processes are considered "active meditations" based on methodical self-inquiries and transform the use of the body as a soothing, grounding mechanism.

A central tenet of Dynamic is that all feelings are an energy. Each energy—or feeling—has its own density, electrical charge, and accompanying behavior, like crying accompanies pain. The energies are on a scale—picture a ladder—where the densest energies are at the bottom, let's say apathy or depression, and as you move up the energetic ladder into feelings like grief, anger, lust, to exemplify a few, the energetic movement increases because it is less dense. I use images when I teach because I find that the mind learns very quickly when it can picture something, and so I invite you to picture bubbles of energy that are condensed and near immobilized at the bottom of the ladder, which is why we are so passive, tired, and foggy when we are depressed. If these "energies" are not released from the body, they accumulate, lump, and atrophy into disorders, syndromes, and ailments. Hence, learning tools and processes to release them are imperative.

For pain or any intense feelings we want to run from, and ones that often stalk and surprise us (like heartbreak, jealousy, and panic), I suggest the following: frame and structure the feeling so that it feels safer to feel it. First, decide on a time to release the feeling. Second, find a place that feels comforting and safe, like a sofa, a meditation corner, or a bench in your garden. Third, once ready, do exactly what Grace suggested: find a way to touch your body to soothe it, such as placing your hand over your heart or holding both hands on your face. This will release the trust hormone oxytocin, and it also comforts the wounded inner child. For feelings that are very intense, I strongly encourage kneeling or lying face down or up to be close to the ground.

Now measure from 1-10, 10 being the most intense and 1 being almost nothing, how strong is your feeling? Once you find your number, create an image of how you will allow the feeling (or the energy bubbles) to leave your body. For example, visualize a valve where your pores release it, or an open door or window through which the energy flows. I personally like combining it with what I've coined as Yes-hales, or long exhales, where I say the word "yesssssssssss" and I visualize the energy leaving throug h my breath. Once you complete a few yes-hales with your image, check back in and measure your number. You are looking for it to have gone down, even if it's a millimeter. As I say in my classes, "We don't do this for free," especially not when it comes to scary, intense feelings; we do this because we want results.

Chapter 3

The Three-Stage Cycle of Narcissistic Abuse

IT'S EXTREMELY PAINFUL AND difficult to get over the betrayal and the cruel acts inflicted by someone who seemed to love you more than anyone. Narcissists have a way of presenting themselves as your ideal partner. They alternate between giving you very good moments (love bombing) and extremely bad ones (discarding). So, you find yourself caught up in this cycle, unconsciously waiting and hoping for the good moments to return. The fact that they never take responsibility for their maliciousness and their total lack of empathy adds to the emotional trauma.

One way to look at this is through the lens of an addictive cycle. The first stage of this cycle is extremely emotionally and physically arousing because there is no other "high" like it, in this case, the "love bombing." What ensues is an unpredictable push/pull pattern that provokes "chasing the original high" and cements the addiction. Realizing that the original high never comes back is an important step. Secondly, ask yourself what you are truly chasing when you chase that high, or what you are seeking to fill?

Consider keeping a journal to track your experiences in the relationship. The need to feel loved can be so acute that we actually gaslight our own memories. "Was it that bad?" "S/he was just hurt," or "I can be very difficult." Write them down with all the details: the name-calling, the silences, the absences, the comparisons...your documentation is an actual tool. If the relationship is beautiful, no harm done, and you are creating a written version of your love story. This is very unlikely with an NPD.

According to NeuroInstincts, individuals with narcissistic traits often engage in a cycle of idealization, devaluation, and discard ("Idealize, Devalue, Discard," n.d.). This vicious cycle strips you of your life-force energy and leaves you feeling devastated and helpless, while the narcissist continues on with their life, seeming totally fine and unaffected by the sabotage of the relationship. It is very common to have feelings of joy and happiness when you start a romantic relationship with someone new. People often describe feeling a sense of euphoria when they begin dating a partner. This is usually referred to as the honeymoon stage in relationships. However, in the narcissistic abuse cycle, this goes to a whole new level.

The Initial Stage of Idealization

In the initial stage, narcissists idealize their new partners and put them on a pedestal. They feel like they have found perfection, and treat you like their newest shiniest toy. This can be mistaken for love as they pour all their affection on their new partner, but unfortunately, this is just an infatuation, kind of like an obsession. The initial stage is very intense and can be overwhelming, but the partner on the receiving end might perceive this as passion and chemistry between the two.

This stage is also known as the love bombing phase, and it provides an emotional high which can be as potent and addictive as drugs like cocaine, heroin, and ecstasy.

The reason why love bombing works so well is that there is a gaping hole to be filled in the victim. This hole tends to be childhood experiences of neglect, intense fear of abandonment, and the "party of one" syndrome, a phrase I've coined to characterize a hard-working child who resolved many things by themselves or for their family and was never mirrored or acknowledged. An actual psychological term is the "parentified child," which is a child who is given adult-like responsibilities prior to when they are ready for them in order to serve the adults or family system that surrounds them. When the narcissist sweeps in and love bombs, that inner child finally has the experience of being seen and valued, and logically, craves more and more validation.

Victims of narcissistic abuse get hooked on this emotional high, and they feel as if they have found their knight in shining armor. At the beginning of the relationship, narcissists fantasize and create an image in their head of their newly found perfect partner, and they truly believe it, as they can be very convincing even with themselves. The thought of finding the perfect partner gives them narcissistic supply, which means boosting their ego as they feel entitled to have the best of everything. The greater the status or quality you offer, the more value you have for them, to first conquer and then destroy.

The Devaluation Stage

As the relationship progresses into a more comfortable rhythm, the narcissist begins to devalue their partner instead of growing closer. They start perceiving their romantic partner as inferior to them, so their narcissistic supply is no longer fueled, and they stop seeing any value in their partner. This results in gaslighting, putting their partner down, intermittently lacking emotional or physical intimacy, withdrawing affection, and blaming their victims for their own mental health issues. Since people with NPD are not able to see their own flaws and imperfections, they end up projecting them onto their significant other to avoid feelings of guilt and shame.

At this stage, the victims will start noticing red flags and realize that something is not right. However, they struggle to end the relationship as by this time, they would have already developed an emotional attachment to the narcissist. Many people who find themselves in this situation start justifying the narcissist's actions and try to convince themselves that they are just going through a rough patch, hoping that they will get their prince charming back. There are countless examples of how a narcissist devalues you; for example, they might show no concern whatsoever for you when you are in a potentially threatening situation. Selfishly so, even though they expect you to attend to their needs even at your own detriment, they are unavailable in times of sickness, distress, or emotional support.

Yes, and like the victim, they have an enormous hole that is never filled and is never explored, so it morphs into an endless black hole that is only temporarily filled by supplying themselves by degrading or abusing another. It is a vampiric distraction from their own empty despair and has addictive mechanics as it is never satisfied; in fact, it grows in tolerance and requires more and more abuse in order to quell their own gaping wound. The vampire metaphor is precise here; energy, time, effort, and attention is getting sucked out of the other.

Also worth noting is the intersection between the victim, or the Empath, and the narcissist who has a similar childhood wound which coalesces into the desire, or rather, the existential begging, to be seen. It is in the response to this wound that marks the difference between the two.

Empaths, who, when unhealed, are perfect partners for the narcissist, will usually understand the narcissist, see their point of view, feel compassion for their childhood or those "rough patches, and secretly believe that at some point the narcissist will reciprocate this empathy. Narcissists, as hard as it is to face, will never reciprocate with authentic empathy.

The Discarding Stage

The third stage of the cycle is the discarding phase, but this does not mean that it's the end of the relationship. Most often, narcissists do not discard permanently, especially if they sense that you can still provide narcissistic supply to them. Every time they discard you and manage to get your attention back, it gives them narcissistic supply as they enjoy getting away with things and pushing people's boundaries. This makes them feel irresistible and more powerful. Narcissists are aware of how painful it is to discard someone, and knowing that they are causing you intense pain, makes them feel satisfied as your emotional pain reaffirms to them how special they are.

The discarding phase is quite dangerous and damaging as victims feel like they are helplessly stuck in a loop. They do not have the strength to leave and go no contact with the narcissist because they find themselves craving their love and affection. Even if they decide to stop all kinds of communication with them, narcissists usually try to creep in to show that they are still there to continue feeling special, admired, and wanted.

When the victims give in and accept the narcissist back, the cycle starts again from the love bombing phase. Narcissists know what they need to do to keep you hooked, so they shower you with compliments or gifts and ideas of your future together, only to take it away again and shatter your dreams.

The discarding stage is the narcissistic secret potion, and it works like a charm. The Empath, or the victim, tends to have enormous abandonment fears and will do almost anything not to be abandoned. The Empath will experience abandonment like a complete loss of the self, as if they do not exist or are completely insignificant, if the narcissist isn't engaging with them. It confirms their worst fear, which is that they are unlovable no matter what they do—"party-of-one" syndrome.

Spoiler alert: the narcissist never truly leaves for this exact reason! Without the Empath, or the victim, to supply them, they feel like they are nothing. It is no surprise narcissists can have multiple lovers for this very reason: they are dependent on various streams of supply because being alone leaves them without a mirror. Again, the intersection of the wound between the Narcissist and Empath is where they are a perfect match... until the Empath or the victim heals! The antidote is to discover that the narcissist collapses without relational supply.

The cycle gets worse the more it repeats itself, and the narcissist projects everything onto the victim. They blame them for everything wrong in the relationship and within themselves. Narcissists twist everything and blame their victims for abuse, lying, and everything they did to victimize themselves. Instead of seeing these behaviors within themselves, they tell their victims that they are the crazy ones, and they portray themselves as the victims of the abuse.

INSIGHTFUL LESSON: Narcissists try to lure you back in, not because they love you, but because they need you for narcissistic supply.

Self-Reflective Exercise:

- Do you recognize this pattern of idealization, devaluation, and discarding in your relationship?
- Can you recall how many times your partner or ex tried to lure you back in with love-bombing, gifts, and promises of a better future together?
- Do you want to continue participating in this abusive cycle? Why?
- Are you still hoping that things will get better? If yes, what makes you believe so?
- What will it take to lose hope that you can make it work?
- What is the scariest thing about leaving your abusive partner?
- What can you do to protect yourself?

Repeat these affirmations at least three times a day for the following thirty days:

- "I love myself and accept myself fully as I am."
- "I deserve to be happy, supported, and loved unconditionally."
- "It is not okay to be devalued and discarded."
- "I only hold space for those who respect me."
- "I prioritize my happiness and well-being over other people's needs."

I tell my clients who are either struggling with an addiction, are code pendent, or can't leave a toxic relationship to do the "End of the Movie" exercise. It is very similar to what Grace has described here, and it requires several failed attempts to change the situation. First, do not see them as "failures," per se, but more as data that establishes a pattern. Once you notice that it is a pattern, you can't relegate it to a random event. Having self-compassion is helpful here because identifying the pattern in this chapter can be a lengthy process; it requires profound introspection and moving past blaming.

The pattern actually reveals your co-participation, which can be hard to see and acknowledge. The exercise is to go to the end of the movie, after he's been called a booty, and is done with sex, or after she's said that she'll never scream at you like that again, or after they say they are changing but ghost you...AGAIN. In these relationships, we keep going back to the start of the relationship; the love swirls, the intimacies, the promises—all forms of future faking. We are chasing the original high. Stop! Picture the end of the movie. How are you left after you come back over and over?

If you're struggling with an addiction—and engaging the narcissist is a relational addiction for sure—picture fully how you feel, where you are left (literally, what room, street, corner), and what you promise yourself. Every. Single. Time. Feel the despair and the loneliness. Go to the end of the movie, not the beginning! As the 12-step adage states, "The definition of insanity is doing the same thing over and over, and expecting different results." Courage—remember, just one change in the pattern begins its dismantling!

Chapter 4

The Four Behavioral Cycles of a Narcissist

EVERYONE HAS ARGUMENTS WITH their romantic partners, but arguing with a narcissist is a totally different ball game. I've lost count of how many times I tried to reason things out with him. After countless letters, long text messages, unanswered calls, and failed attempts to have logical and fact-based debates, I had finally given up. I felt like I was always on edge, and I could never feel completely relaxed, as I was always expecting something to come up. Even events which were supposed to be joyful and entertaining turned into painful memories and disappointing outcomes.

An argument with a narcissist follows the same pattern. It's a toxic, vicious cycle that keeps repeating itself until you decide that you have had enough. Bringing this pattern to your awareness will make it easier for you to break the cycle and decide to leave the abusive relationship.

Ego Feels Threatened

As soon as an upsetting event occurs, no matter how small and irrelevant it is, narcissists feel threatened due to their unrealistic expectations and perfectionism. Anything could trigger this response, for example, feeling rejected or unappreciated in some way, disapproval at work, embarrassment in a social setting, jealousy of others, or feeling neglected and disrespected. Narcissists tend to obsess and get upset over the same frivolous things, regardless of whether the issue is real or imagined. They keep bringing up the same argument, hold grudges, and struggle to move forward and let things go.

Narcissistic supply has at its core a sadistic need to fill an abyss that is only filled momentarily by the complete demeaning of another. It may seem strange from the outside, but inflicting cruelty upon another is the only way they feel like they exist. On a grander scale, this phenomenon occurs in families, cults, schools, offices, and nations. One group sadistically demeans another group to gratify their sense of inadequacy.

It's logical, really: someone or a group that feels fulfilled or content with who they are and has a self-affirming mirror has no need to inflict pain upon another. In fact, they have no need to be at war with another, because they have an internal peace in their home, i.e., their families, countries, or self. Narcissism and the need to prove superiority and control the power dynamics are at the forefront of all wars. And as we know from history, war can become an obsessive pursuit.

Once, I was heading out of our apartment for a coffee date with a friend of mine. As I was walking down the stairs, I was looking for a €50 note that I was sure I had put in my purse. I went back to our apartment and asked him if he had seen the €50 note, and he told me that he hadn't seen it. I thought I had lost it, so I continued with my day and went out to meet my friend.

The following morning, he came up to me with a smile on his face, telling me that he had found a €50 note outside our apartment. I got excited that he had found it, and I asked him to return it to me. He immediately got defensive and told me how rude I was for asking him for money, which he had found. I was shocked! Did he forget what I had told him the day before? I reminded him of our conversation on the previous day before I went out to meet my friend. But he insisted that he should keep the money because I had no proof whatsoever that the money was mine. I fought back, I was tired of being submissive all the time, and his ego did not like that!

Engaging in Abusive Behavior

My reluctance to be submissive did not go down well with him. The following hours were filled with rage and aggression. He demanded that I apologize to him and that if I wanted my money back, I should get down on my knees and beg him for it.

This moment is extremely important: as the narcissist feels that his or her victim is gaining independence or a sense of self, they will impose greater punishments and/or sadistic requests like this one. Why is this important? Because as they start to feel like they no longer have a hold on the person, they may get more violent psychologically, physically, and emotionally.

A warning here: the moment of regaining self-control and gaining independence can also be a very dangerous moment because it undergirds and shocks the narcissist. At this juncture is when we see an increase in domestic abuse, all-out wars raged during custody battles, smear campaigns, and even homicide. Strategy is required: get physical, emotional, and spiritual support in the forms of community, protection, and evidence. There is more support today than ever. Do not be discouraged to break free—support, strategy, and wisdom are your essential tools here.

I couldn't believe what was coming out of his mouth. I felt nauseous, and I remember saying to myself, *"Oh God, this is sick, he really is a psycho, and I don't want to participate in this crazy drama anymore!"* By that time, I knew what he was capable of, yet he still managed to surprise me.

A beautiful glimpse of the healed inner self! Her body reminds her by feeling sick that sickness is in her midst, and she finally is giving his behavior a place: back to himself!

Narcissists are bullies; they are incapable of managing their emotions, especially when their ego feels threatened. His ego couldn't accept the fact that I was rising above him. So, to try to gain his power back over me, he immediately started engaging in abusive behavior.

Someone who always needs to be right or to always win—key word is always—can be an early sign to catch. Even if you are in the love bombing stage, notice if he needs to be right or needs to win all discussions with others.

He tried to make me feel small so his ego could feel superior again. Narcissists know how to trigger you and which buttons to push. Their abuse is specifically targeted to exploit your weaknesses. They attack your self-esteem by verbal belittling and excessive criticism to wear you out, leaving you feeling useless and unworthy. This kind of behavior destroys your self-esteem, and eventually, you end up forgetting your own positive qualities and abilities as they rob you of your self-worth.

What I am suspecting here is that Grace's partner may have felt threatened about her going out with a friend for coffee because it means that she has a life without him which weakens his power over her. This is why Narcissists strategically isolate their victims. In order to re-establish the power dynamic, he had to punish her by withholding the money and belittling her. Even if this wasn't the case in this instance, this is a classic tactic wherein the Narcissist feels like he won and "showed" who dictates the terms of engagement.

Playing the Victim

His attempt to manipulate me failed miserably this time. I refused to bow down to him and ask him for something that was mine in the first place. As usual, he followed the same predictable pattern and started blaming me for everything that was wrong in his life. He told me how much he hated me because I brought out the worst in him. And he made me believe that he never had any arguments with anyone else because I was the problem. I was the one to blame for *everything*.

I'm sure you've realized by now that narcissists have a way of twisting facts and circumstances to portray themselves as the victims. I fell for his manipulative techniques many times, and I used to end up feeling guilty for things I didn't do. Feelings of remorse and guilt pushed me to accept this warped perception, and I just wanted to do something to improve our relationship. To resolve the situation, I ended up begging him for forgiveness and accepted responsibility and blame for what had happened.

Here, they are "emotionally molesting" Grace by using guilt. The strategic use of fear, shame, and guilt is emotional molestation because it pulls on the victim, child, or Empath's natural instinct not to want to hurt them. This is a human instinct, by the way, to not want to cause damage, especially when someone is claiming to be hurt.

Feeling Empowered

He got exactly what he wanted! Accepting responsibility for what happened leaves narcissists feeling empowered. This kind of behavior reaffirms to them that they are superior and that they are always right about things. Unknowingly, I was providing him with narcissistic supply, and the weaker I got, the stronger his ego grew. Back then, I didn't realize that being submissive was not resolving the issue, but was actually making it worse.

The Empath is naturally hardwired to "resolve" and "harmonize," and this natural tendency is strategically exploited by the NPD, over and over. Submission is also a mammalian instinct to appease a dominant figure. The twist here, as Grace noted, is that it leads to more dominance, and in this relational model, the one with self-respect becomes the stronger one.

Narcissists are like kids. Just like a toddler learns that throwing a tantrum will get his mother to buy him a second ice-cream, narcissists learn that engaging in abusive behavior will drive their victims to surrender. My submission reaffirmed to him that the next time something doesn't go his way, he knows what he needs to do to get whatever he wants.

Most victims repeatedly make the same mistakes I did. They believe that they can get the narcissist to see their point of view and reason things out. They try to explain themselves and bring up evidence to sustain their arguments.

Let's provide some hope here: this is a natural human response, and with people who are reasonable and meet the minimum standard of human care, seeing another's point of view, receiving explanations, and listening to each other works! Often, the world of the narcissist can seem like the only world, but as one heals, there is a world of mutual care, feedback, and respectful resolution out there. Sadly, and yes, very sadly, this is not the case with the NPD because of their inability to empathize. It doesn't make sense to go to a well that doesn't provide water. Reciprocity is a key ingredient to a healthy relationship.

What they fail to realize is that you cannot reason things out with a narcissist. A person who suffers from a narcissistic personality disorder is highly unlikely to admit to any wrongdoing, as it is against their true nature. The four behavioral cycles repeat themselves each time the ego feels threatened. It starts the same way, and it ends the same way, leaving you feeling guilty, ashamed, confused, and miserable.

How to Spot the Abusive Behavior of a Narcissist

When you try to argue with a narcissist, you always end up having the same outcome, and that involves feeling hurt, misunderstood, isolated, and confused. Their manipulative techniques can be hard to identify as they are so subtle, yet extremely effective. Learning about these gaslighting techniques and what to look for can help you to take a step back and rethink your next move the next time you have an argument with the narcissist.

Manipulative gaslighting techniques usually involve the following behaviors:

Guilt-Tripping

Narcissists try to make you feel guilty for your actions and decisions to get what they want. They try to make you feel ashamed, even when you try to stand up for yourself or to protect yourself. Their objective is to make you feel guilty, so you end up apologizing and surrendering to what they want.

This is what I have coined "emotional molestation," and it also includes using fear and shame.

Lying

To avoid taking responsibility or taking the blame for their unethical behaviors, narcissists lie to control and persuade others. They will do just about anything to avoid paying the consequences for their actions.

Projection

Narcissists do this all the time. They project their own wrongdoing on others and blame someone else for their actions. Projection can take form in many different ways, and it makes others feel responsible for their actions.

Lying and projecting go hand in hand in that the narcissist is constantly lying to themselves and desperately needs others on whom to project their lies. Having any look at their internal experience is too painful, so everything, everything must be spewed outside of themselves.

Love-Bombing

This is not the same as showing honest affection towards someone. Love bombing is a manipulative technique where narcissists shower you with excessive attention, affection, gifts, compliments, or false promises. Their intention is not genuine as their motive is to manipulate you to get what they want.

Changing Expectations

Narcissists enjoy seeing other people trying hard to please them. They change their expectations to keep you constantly working hard to please them. Despite your successes, they don't acknowledge your efforts, leaving you feeling exhausted and frustrated.

I call this "hoop jumping." Hoop jumping takes a while to recognize because it is usually distracted by the promise of something. "If you do this, you'll get that." "We'll get married and have babies, but right now..." "If you do this or tolerate this (like never getting a job or never paying or raging explosions), I'll stay with you..."

It's a classic donkey-and-carrot scenario, and can be quite mesmerizing because it engages powerful fantasies of a "fake future." I put love bombing and hoop jumping under the broader category of "mirage," and it takes a while to see past the mirage. One way to recognize hoop jumping and looking beyond the mirage is to look at the actual concrete evidence. Ask questions like "How long has he or she promised this?" "Does he or she give me what I want after I jump the hoops?" "Is there always a next hoop to jump?" "How much time has passed since they first promised this?" are very good questions that shatter the mirage.

Withdrawal/Silent Treatment

Withdrawal is a form of emotional manipulation when the narcissist punishes you by withholding affection and intimacy from you. This kind of manipulation causes a power imbalance in the relationship. They also use the silent treatment to punish you by ignoring you. This leaves you craving their attention and validation.

Withdrawal, silent treatment, and walking away behaviors activate the abandonment fear and wound in the child, wounded Empath, or victim. It is a very intense experience that can collapse unhealed people into cycles of great, destructive shame.

Comparison

Narcissists enjoy making their partners feel insecure by comparing them to others. They provoke feelings of unworthiness and blame them for not being good enough for them. This demoralizes their victims and makes them feel like they cannot live up to their standards.

Triangulation

To invalidate your feelings and reactions to their abusive behavior, narcissists involve others who are also influenced by them. Their objective is to validate their point of view and evoke uncertainty in you. They want you to doubt your feelings, thoughts, and perceptions so you become more susceptible to abuse.

I describe comparison and triangulation as the "divide and conquer" strategy that occurs often in families. The abusive narcissistic parent will pit one sibling against another with the use of superior/inferior comparisons. The child who feels preferred feels seen and special, but also feels confused because it's at the expense of their sibling. The favor can also change at the drop of a dime, and the other sibling is preferred (expectation changing). This places the family in a state of competition and war with an increasing need to gain the narcissistic parent's favor. The narcissist has thus divided and conquered.

This strategy can also be translated to the narcissist who is involved in another relationship or is married. They will demean or criticize the spouse to the new person while love bombing them. The new person will feel special and seen for their good traits and will feel like they are "winning" against the partner or spouse. Grace described this exact scenario when she first met her narcissistic abuser. Underneath this divide and conquer strategy, trust is eroding, and stability feels fragile. Everyone unconsciously becomes a chess piece, and fear of losing favor keeps the game going. This is a precise definition of nations at war and strategies around alliances and power dynamics.

INSIGHTFUL LESSON: A narcissist will never validate your feelings. You don't need anyone to tell you that what you're feeling or experiencing is true. you are enough.

Self-Reflective Exercise:

- Do you struggle to validate your own feelings?
- Do you have a tendency to ask others to validate what you're feeling or experiencing?
- Do you find yourself doubting whether your perceptions or reactions are real or appropriate?
- Are you constantly trying to get the narcissist to see your point of view, but end up feeling exhausted and frustrated?

Validating Your Own Feelings & Experiences

Start writing down your thoughts, feelings, and experiences in a journal. After you've finished writing, write down the following affirmations:

- "I acknowledge and accept my feelings without judgment."
- "I validate my own feelings and experiences."
- "I know what's right and wrong."

Acknowledge and accept your feelings with self-compassion and without judgment. It's *okay* to feel this way. Remember that everything will pass and that this is only temporary.

Imagine that a dear friend of yours was going through the same situation and came asking you for advice. What would you tell her?

When I teach Dynamic, I encourage students to approach their feelings mechanically or technically. I suggest this because sometimes feelings can be so horrific, like when trauma-triggered, or overwhelming, like during a panic attack, that if we approach them mechanically or visually (like the energetic bubbles example), we can begin to befriend them.

An exercise I use to validate feelings is the "Now Feeling" exercise, which I also consider a meditation because it emphasizes the now moment. Take a piece of paper and divide it into 3 columns. At the top of the first column, ask yourself, "What is my now feeling?." Refrain from judging or analyzing, and move through it at a fast-ISH pace because this exercise is meant to be technical, per se, to make it less intimidating. Your answer may be "enraged," then add a number next to it (from 1-10 measurement). Quickly ask again, "What is my now feeling?" The answer may be "still enraged," and add your number.

Keep going until you fill all 3 columns. Let's say you have 4 "enraged" in a row, you will find that a new feeling will pop...like "devastated," "scared," and keep going. The quick pace, and number measurements circumvent self-judgement and/or rabbit hole impulses. Keep going all the way to the end of the 3rd column. When I do this with my clients, I am looking for inevitably more vulnerable or more buried feelings.

I ask, "What pops?" What I mean by that is, "What is the unconscious popping up?" If we just keep asking the question over and over, "What is my now feeling?" it will pop up the unconscious, and that's what we want to unearth in order to untangle the pattern.

Beautiful, isn't it? Healing is beautiful. You are not alone in this work, and it is time for you to read this book.

Chapter 5

The Symptoms of Narcissistic Abuse

When I was going through hell with my ex, I wasn't aware that I was a victim of domestic violence, which is ironic considering the fact that I had spent eight years working in the Family Court on cases pertaining to domestic violence. It had never occurred to me that one day I would be one of those victims.

Psychologically, I would define this as an unconscious behavior, where Grace is working in a field where she needs help. This is an unconscious request. If Grace had come into my office, I would have investigated her choice of career or work because we can often find childhood underpinnings that seem dormant. Spiritually, this is the law of attraction at work. The law of attraction is always at play, whether we want it to be or not. And, whether we are aware of it or not, our external life is a mirror to our internal world. Look around your external world and ask yourself, "How is this showing me something about myself?"

Throughout our relationship, I had normalized his abusive behavior. Even though I knew he was not treating me well, I denied the severity of the circumstances. The first time I realized that I was a victim of domestic violence was three years into the relationship, when we were living together. An article popped up on my news feed speaking about different forms of abuse and domestic violence. The article highlighted that emotional and verbal abuse were also criminal offenses that fell under the category of domestic violence.

I showed him the article, and I foolishly thought that he would back down and apologize for his behavior. Instead, he denied that he had ever hurt me in any way and accused me of trying to put him in jail for nothing. The argument escalated quickly, even though I had tried to explain to him that I had no intention of filing a police report and taking him to court.

Once again, I was punished with hateful words for hours on end, followed by the silent treatment for the whole week. Being isolated in my own house gave me space and time to reflect on what was happening. I realize now how knowledge gave me the power and confidence to stand up for myself. If only I had known from the very beginning that what he was doing to me was unacceptable and illegal, I believe that my story would have turned out differently.

Kudos, Grace! And today we have so much information and support available for healing, including this book. In my work and throughout the history of mankind, we see that where humans feel most alone, most susceptible, most impoverished, and hence, can be the most enslaved, is in our not knowing. It is no coincidence that the start of any dictatorship, enslavement, or domination of another group begins with the burning of books, isolation, and the collapse of information. When we don't know, we are confused and scared, and thus, we can be steered more easily, even to our own demise. Knowledge is power.

It was difficult to accept that I was a victim of domestic violence. I was a well-educated young woman, and I felt ashamed of myself for not realizing what was happening to me. But I was too busy focusing on how to please him and make things work.

What Grace is describing here is a common shame: why does someone who may come from a "good family," who is educated, and seems psychologically aware, fall into these abusive relationships? Why do people smoke in an era where data shows it's cancerous? Why do people eat the second pizza when they are already nearing 300 pounds? Why do we engage in these behaviors and relationships when we should know better?

It's because of the Triune brain: the executive brain, the limbic brain, and the reptilian brain. Even though they collaborate, and all three serve survival purposes, they each have different functions, memories, and drives. In other words, having a high IQ or being well educated (executive brain functions) does not mean that we are emotionally sound and may have even used our intellectual prowess as a defense for deep emotional wounds (limbic brain functions). Our limbic brain runs the show very often when it comes to addictions, compulsions, and relational dysfunctions, and therein is where the deep work is done through therapy and meditation.

When you're in a relationship with a narcissist, it's easy to get stuck in a loop where you keep trying to change the narcissist's behavior. I tried everything and nothing worked. At some point, I tricked myself into believing that if I mirrored his behavior and gave him a taste of his own medicine, things would change. Of course, that didn't work either, and I found myself always feeling on edge, anticipating his next move, so I could be prepared for it. I kept trying to force the relationship in a direction, and it cost me my health. I felt extremely stressed and depressed, I lost interest in everything and my entire being was consumed by anxiously trying to figure out how to make things better. My chronic anxiety started to show, and friends and colleagues couldn't help but notice that something was very wrong with me. One morning, I was at the office staring blankly outside the window. A colleague of mine who was in her mid-50s looked at me and commented on how old I looked.

Along the path of dysfunctional relationships, there are spectators who see it happening and gossip, and there are what I like to call "the earth angels" who appear and kindly say something, even when you are not likely to hear it. These earth angels will say, "Something is changing in you—are you okay?" "You look older or sickly—are you okay?" "You don't seem like yourself, you're not as joyful—are you okay? "

More often than not, we respond defensively or ignore it, but these are moments when your inner being will perk up and feel validated. What you decide to do with those comments is what determines your trajectory. In any case, know that your higher self, higher power, or inner being is always trying to get your attention. You will remember these earth angels later with great affection, as disturbing as they may feel in the moment.

I was speechless. A middle-aged woman had remarked on how old I looked, and I was only 27 years old! I remember taking my mobile phone and looking at my reflection. She was right! I did look old, like a wilted flower drained of life force and energy.

The severe anxiety was eating me from the inside. I looked pale, skinny and weak. I started smoking weed from day to night to numb the pain and manage my anxiety. As soon as I woke up, I used to take a few hits, and the last thing I did before going to bed was smoke a big joint to help me pass out. Smoking weed helped me numb the pain, but at some point, it just wasn't enough. No matter how much I tried to escape reality, the pain was still there. I tried to run away from the pain and from my biggest fears, but looking back now, I know that the only way to free myself from the pain was to end the relationship and remove him from my life.

As I continued researching this personality disorder throughout our relationship, I realized that I had developed narcissistic abuse syndrome. My self-esteem and my physical and mental well-being were adversely affected. I felt worthless and unloved, and I was always trying to be better. In this chapter, I explain the signs and symptoms of narcissistic abuse. If you notice some of these symptoms, *run away*! It's a sign that you're dealing with an emotional predator.

Walking on Eggshells

You know what it feels like when your abuser gets triggered, and you know that he or she has a short temper. So you start being extra careful with how you talk and act around the narcissist. The problem is that narcissists always find something to complain about, so avoiding triggering situations doesn't make the problem go away. I remember I was always on edge in his presence. I could never relax and feel at ease, neither when we were alone, nor when we were socializing with friends and family. God forbid someone would joke with him or put him in an uncomfortable situation. I never lowered my guard and was always trying to protect his fragile ego, acting as a mediator between him and other people. Otherwise, I knew I would have to pay the consequences.

Narcissists treat you like their emotional punching bag. So, you end up feeling perpetually anxious about provoking or confronting the narcissist, and you start becoming invisible or wanting to be invisible. This gives them even more space to continue engaging in abusive behavior as they know that you won't fight back.

This is an example of the "walking dead syndrome" I described earlier, marked by the glazed-over or zombie look. The defensive strategy here is to get smaller and smaller, or to exist less and less, in order not to attract the abuser. Another example of this—in an opposite way but with the same hope—is when someone who has been or is being sexually abused gains more and more weight. The hope is, "Maybe I won't be seen or attract any more attention."

In both scenarios, there's a desperation to become invisible to the abuser. I have seen children become selectively mute, wives literally lose their ability to find words, and husbands who eat themselves into a heart attack, to not engage the NPD, all along screaming for help. These symptoms are all addressed as other clinical disorders, unless we observe them from a family systems perspective, where we can identify the holistic systemic dynamics of living with an NPD.

By continuing to pretend that everything is okay around the narcissist, you fail to be true to yourself and neglect your needs. In time, you lose your personality as a result of wearing a mask for a long time, and you end up losing yourself along the way.

Loss of Self-Worth

Our brains learn by repetition as neural pathways increase and get stronger the more we practice something, until it becomes our new normal. The same goes for verbal abuse and insulting nicknames. Eventually, you start believing the belittling comments about yourself. You find yourself questioning whether you're actually good at anything. And the positive qualities that you once knew you had start fading out of your memory.

This is an actual war tactic: by demeaning the enemy, by calling the enemy names, by seeing them as less than human, it is easier to abuse, torture, or kill them. It actually dehumanizes both the perpetrator and the victim and goes against our core human characteristic to empathize or care about another. It also serves to subjugate and create "learned helplessness," as I described earlier. The will to fight back is eroded. So it's always amazing and uplifting when our inner being—including in cases of war—fights back! I like to track and mark these times as moments of spiritual revolution. It is so important to honor these times as moments when your inner being was helping you stay alive, literally and metaphorically.

Being constantly reminded of how worthless you are destroys your self-esteem and can result in self-hatred and self-harm. Loss of self-worth and self-respect is not always that obvious, though. In my case, I had tricked myself into believing that I respected myself, as I used to call him out on his lies and erratic behavior. I fought hard to set boundaries and gave him countless ultimatums. What I failed to realize was that by complaining about something, I didn't have any control over the situation or his behavior.

By sticking around, I was tolerating the abuse. I was complaining, but I was still allowing it to happen. Throughout my journey of transformation, I learned what it meant to really love and respect yourself. And I realized that it didn't make sense to give my precious time and energy to someone who didn't and couldn't appreciate it. Why should you stay begging someone to see your worth when there are so many others who can do so effortlessly?

But here's a hard pill to swallow: this won't happen until you do the inner work. You cannot attract people who genuinely value you if, at your core, you don't truly value yourself. Your external reality is not random—it is a direct reflection of your unconscious beliefs, playing out over and over again until you bring awareness to them.

Understanding this is everything. If you don't recognize the role your inner world plays in shaping your outer experiences, you will continue to find yourself in the same painful patterns, wondering why things never seem to change. I know this because I was there too. At first, I couldn't see that I didn't fully value myself. It was an unconscious belief running my life, subtly influencing the people I attracted and the experiences I had. But through painful realizations, mindfulness practices, and deep work in psychotherapy, this truth was finally brought to the surface.

That's why inner work isn't just important—it's essential. Until you shift your internal world, your external reality will continue to reflect the same patterns. But the moment you begin to transform within, the world around you will start to shift in ways you never imagined.

Always Feeling Like You've Done Something Wrong

Trying to get a narcissist to admit that they've done something wrong is bound to fail and end in disappointment. For example, you might call them out on cheating, and they immediately switch to a defensive state. Before you know it, the situation escalates quickly, and all of a sudden, you end up being shamed for doubting their loyalty. They accuse you of paranoia, and shame you for snooping around through their things. They have a way of twisting the argument and deflecting the attention on something you've done so they can scold you and punish you.

I remember one particular event when we were living together. It was one of those days when we had spent the whole day arguing. After endless hours of arguing, it was time for bed. We were going to start watching something on Netflix, but he immediately tried to start having sex with me. I was still feeling broken and shaken after all the hateful words that had just come out of his mouth. So, I told him that I needed some time to calm down, and I insisted on watching a movie. He felt rejected, and you know that rejection doesn't go down very well with narcissists. To try and have his way with me, he threatened me that if I didn't satisfy his needs whenever he pleased, then I'm the one to blame if he starts seeking other women. I felt helpless and that no matter what I did, even when I tried to protect myself, I felt like I was doing something wrong.

Foolishly so, I tried to make it up to him, so the next day I decided to cook him a nice dinner. I rushed to the grocery store as soon as he left for work, and I bought all his favorite ingredients. Everything needed to be perfect! I slaved around in the kitchen all day and prepared a three-course meal for him. I was excited! Dinner was ready right on time, and as soon as he returned home, I greeted him with a big smile on my face. The moment he came in, he could sense my desperate need for his validation. He started looking around in the kitchen, inspecting what I had cooked for him. At first, he seemed pleased until he noticed that I didn't use his favorite type of olive oil in the recipe. Hell broke loose.

The following hours were filled with rage and degrading comments. He mocked me and insulted me by calling me all sorts of names. He took joy from reminding me how incompetent and useless I was to him. My heart was shattered into pieces, and I felt so stupid for choosing the incorrect olive oil. I felt so close to making him happy, and I was angry at myself for screwing up again by choosing the wrong ingredient! After he tired himself out, he took the food from the kitchen and locked himself in our main bedroom. He ignored me throughout the whole week and punished me with the silent treatment. Ironically enough, he ate all the food. Looking back at this memory as I'm writing this book, I find myself laughing at how silly his complaint sounds. I realize how his reaction was completely out of proportion and how monumental those "mistakes" seem.

It is important to remember here that who shows up wanting to please the narcissist, is the inner child. This correlates to a childhood wound of wanting to make a parent or a caregiver happy, and children do this all the time. The wish is that if they are able to make the caregiver happy—whether it be that the caregiver is overworked, depressed, always complaining, or abusive—the child will finally get loving parenting.

Let me repeat, the child feels that if they are able to make the caregiver happy by solving the problem, by being funny, by being good, by cleaning the house, etc., the caregiver will finally have the wherewithal to parent the child. This creates the "parentified child." A child who takes on the adult role of a parent in order to get parenting. This attempt—and many others—to make the narcissist happy, along with it being a normal, human behavior to want our loved ones to be happy, is an attempt to get love back. The psychological pattern or formula is "if I make them happy, then they will finally..."

Back then, I fell for his manipulative tricks and tried harder to please him and to feel good enough. Eventually, I started feeling grateful that he was willing to stay with someone like me, who was always making mistakes. The feeling of unworthiness stuck with me even after ending the relationship. And the thought of not being able to do anything right became ingrained in my subconscious as an inner core belief.

Dissociation as a Coping Mechanism

At the end of my relationship, I couldn't help but notice how disconnected I felt from my emotions. It was quite scary as I had never felt this way before. I couldn't feel anything, neither joy nor sadness. I just felt numb. No matter what I tried to do, I couldn't get myself to experience any kind of emotion. At first, I didn't realize what was happening, but then I realized that I was trying so hard to numb the pain that it finally worked to a certain extent. I remember doing research about it to try to "fix myself." I didn't want to stay emotionally numb forever, and it took me months to start feeling something again.

Through research, I had learned that dissociation describes a type of psychological disconnect where victims of abuse check out from their reality to numb the emotional pain. Instead of fighting or running from a situation, a person retreats into their mind and completely detaches from the situation to protect themselves from overwhelming stress. This distorts your experience of identity, memory, and consciousness, and negatively affects your self-awareness and perception of your environment.

This kind of coping mechanism is how you start approaching life in general because it's a way of escaping from your current reality. To avoid dealing with the full terror of your circumstances, your brain finds ways to emotionally block out the impact of your pain.

This is a beautiful description of disassociation, and I like to add that it is a beautiful protective mechanism from our inner being or our higher power to help us leave a moment of complete terror, as in the case of physical, sexual, or emotional abuse. As children, dissociation serves as a protective mechanism against horror. As in all defense mechanisms, and as Grace precisely depicts here, once it becomes a psychological habit and a way of being, it can wreak havoc on adult relationships. Defense mechanisms originally appeared to help us, but if left unchecked and unprocessed, they will stalk our relational future. Compassionate self-reflection and self-observation are the defense detanglers, and psychotherapy, holistic coaching, and mediation are good sources for this work.

Thankfully, this process is reversible, but it requires a great deal of patience, self-compassion, and support from someone who can guide you along your process of healing.

I really had to work hard to connect with myself and strengthen my mind-body connection. Self-awareness was an essential element in my healing process as I needed to be aware of what was happening within me to understand what I was going through on a psychological level.

Psychosomatic Symptoms

Stress can kill you, literally! The body cannot tell the difference between legitimate fear, where your survival is at risk, and whether you're just scared and distressed on a psychological level. According to the American Psychological Association (APA), chronic stress can have detrimental effects on both physical and mental health ("Chronic Stress," 2014). Prolonged exposure to abuse can trigger physiological symptoms as your emotional trauma starts manifesting as a sickness in your body and disrupts physiological functioning. The brain activates involuntary nervous and biochemical responses, which can result in dysfunction or structural damage in physical organs.

Some of the most common symptoms are changes in appetite, nausea and gastrointestinal distress, muscle aches, restlessness, panic attacks, nervousness, insomnia, and fatigue. As a natural reaction to stress, your adrenal glands release the hormone cortisol into your bloodstream. Cortisol increases your heart rate and blood pressure as part of the fight-or-flight response, a survival instinct that evolved with us for thousands of years.

Brain fog is also a common symptom among victims of narcissistic abuse, which is a result of elevated cortisol levels in your system. So, if you have been having trouble focusing and lack mental clarity, it could be a result of high cortisol levels due to severe stress. Increased cortisol can hamper your immune system, making you weaker and more susceptible to getting sick. You might also notice that you have gained or lost a significant amount of weight and experienced physical symptoms of premature aging. This process is known as the telomere effect, where cortisol accelerates the aging process.

I love this whole section and the fact that in our current society, people are finally catching on to the idea that mind, body, heart, and spirit are multiple operating systems encased in one larger unified whole wherein each impacts the other. Physical symptomatology can have direct emotional, mental, and spiritual antecedents and can be evaluated through that lens. A holistic counselor (like me) or a coach will diagnose everything that happens to you physically via the lens of an internal cause. The body is constantly sending us messages, so listening and investigating are key.

Complex Post-Traumatic Stress Disorder

Also known as C-PTSD, this is a psychological disorder that develops due to a series of traumatic events, where victims feel trapped with no chance of escape. You feel powerless and become increasingly submissive to your abuser. When you try to explain what you are going through, you find it difficult to pinpoint exactly what it is. This is due to the fact that narcissists are able to twist reality to avoid taking responsibility for their actions. Let's have a look at the most common symptoms of C-PTSD:

- Difficulty managing emotions
- Depression
- Thoughts of self-harm

- Repressed memories of traumatic events
- Feelings of shame and guilt
- A sense of distrust and hopelessness
- Flashbacks
- Hypervigilance
- Dissociation

The difference between Complex Post-Traumatic Disorder and Simple Post-Traumatic Disorder (or just PTSD) is that Complex Post-Traumatic Disorder includes repetitive trauma over an extended period of time. Simple PTSD is a one-case scenario, as in experiencing a car accident or losing a limb unexpectedly. Both have intense psychological consequences, but C-PTSD takes longer to heal because it lasts for a longer period of time with multiple, repetitive episodes. A word of encouragement: now more than ever, there are comprehensive modalities that help in the healing of C-PTSD. The word is out, and the good news is here that through a process called neuroplasticity—which is the neuroscientific finding that even as traumatized adults we can heal through new experiences—we can find a future with possibilities.

When you develop C-PTSD, initially, you might deny the abuse as a survival mechanism to avoid facing the painful emotions that you are going through. You might also rationalize and justify the abuser's behavior, and try to convince yourself and those around you that the narcissist is not that bad. However, deep down in your heart, you know that something is not right, but you try to silence your own conscience. According to PsychCentral, there are certain signs that can indicate if someone is in denial about their trauma ("Denial of Trauma Signs," n.d.).

These sound like:

- "Everything is fine. I'm OK, really don't worry about me."
- "I'm sure that everyone has these kinds of problems."
- "It's not a big deal, he said he's sorry and that he will make it up to me."
- "It's not that bad, you can't call it trauma."
- "That's not what happened to me."
- "I'm strong and I can deal with this by myself."
- "I'd rather not think about it too much."
- "I overreacted, it wasn't that bad after all."

If this sounds like you or you are familiar with these symptoms, show up for yourself and seek the support you need to process your emotions and start healing. Denial might seem like a quick fix for the problem. However, the only way to really be free from suffering is to allow yourself to feel your emotions so you can address them. Once you get to the other side of healing, you will be able to experience a sense of inner peace and wholeness within yourself.

Sense of Mistrust

This is something I personally struggled with for a very long time. Not only did I lose my sense of trust in others, but also in myself. Having someone deny your experiences and emotions day in and day out leaves you incapable of trusting your own emotions and perceptions.

Narcissists are masters of denial and manipulation, and they have a way of making you feel that your feelings and experiences are invalid. Being constantly lied to, while having your version of the story denied at all times, is detrimental to your emotional health. You start believing that you cannot trust what you are experiencing, and you continuously push your feelings down instead of addressing them.

Moreover, when you realize that the person you once trusted had malicious intentions, you find yourself feeling anxious and doubtful of other people's intentions. Every person becomes a potential threat, and you become hypervigilant, which leaves you feeling overwhelmed with stress and anxiety. Distrusting others also makes it harder to form intimate connections and authentic relationships, including friendships.

The sense of mistrust showed up in every aspect of my life. I felt paralyzed and struggled to make any kind of decision for myself. It took me years to learn how to trust myself again. I invested my time and energy in reconnecting to my true self and strengthening my sense of intuition. I wanted to make sure that before I started trusting others again, I could trust my sense of judgment to protect myself from getting hurt again.

There is something so humanly profound about what Grace is saying here. Trust is at the very heart of feeling securely attached to a parent. Trust implies safety, and safety provides us with the ability to explore and expand beyond the perimeters of what is known. When a child feels securely attached to their caregiver, they feel safe enough to explore the world around them. They know that making mistakes is part of the process, and they can come back to the safe haven of their loving caregiver's arms.

This stands true to trusting oneself. If we have a safe relationship with our SELF, if we have the compassion to allow for mistakes and growth, we can fully expand and evolve into our best or highest selves. When we lose trust in another or in our SELF, we lose a key tenet of human existence and the ability to compassionately care. When trust is robbed from us, what is usurped is our compassionate care for ourselves and others, and it is replaced with a constant sense of danger; war thus follows. It is clear and essential: it behooves us to do this work of self-trust, self-love, and self-compassion in order for us to remain in relationship with others and the world. The narcissist engenders the exact opposite outcome.

Deciding to commit to myself and to work on the relationship with myself was the best decision I ever made. The process of healing and reconnecting with my true essence helped me find my inner strength and access my inner wisdom. For the first time in my life, I felt guided by my own intuition, which gave me the courage to find my way back in society.

INSIGHTFUL LESSON: The most important relationship to work on is the relationship with yourself.

Nobody deserves to stay in an emotionally abusive relationship. If you are currently in an abusive relationship of any kind, keep in mind that you are not alone. There are many survivors who managed to overcome it. You don't have to feel ashamed that you found yourself in this situation. This kind of psychological torment is not exclusive to any gender, culture, social class, or religion. Don't be scared to reach out for help if you are experiencing any of these symptoms.

It is not easy to leave an abusive relationship due to the intense effects of trauma and the prevalent sense of helplessness and hopelessness. Find the strength within you and remind yourself that it is, in fact, possible to leave and begin the journey of healing. Even though recovering from the abuse is challenging, it is well worth paving the path to freedom. One day, you will be free from the trauma, and you will become stronger and more resilient with a strong sense of empowerment: "Like the lotus flower that blooms out of mud, we shall embrace our painful experiences, because they will help us grow and transform into our most beautiful authentic self."

Emotional Freedom Technique

According to EFT International, EFT tapping is a technique that combines acupressure with psychology to address emotional and physical issues ("What is EFT Tapping?" n.d.).

This technique was introduced back in the 1990s by Gary Craig. It's a form of psychological acupressure to reduce physical and emotional pain.

Use this EFT tapping technique when you feel anxious, stressed, or overwhelmed with emotions.

Step 1: Identify and label your emotion.

Step 2: Rank the intensity of the emotion on a scale of 1-10, with 10 being the most intense.

Step 3: Choose a self-love and self-acceptance phrase that you will repeat to yourself while tapping on different body points. Ex: "Even though I feel hurt and rejected, I love myself and I accept myself completely."

Step 4: Use two or more fingertips and start tapping on these specific points on your body. Tap five times on each point while repeating the chosen phrase.

Follow this sequence while tapping:

1. **Top of the head:** Directly in the center of the crown of your head.
2. **Beginning of the eyebrows:** The beginning of your eyebrows, just above the side of your nose.
3. **Side of the eyes:** At the outside corner of your eyes on the bone.
4. **Under the eyes:** On the bone under your eyes.
5. **Under the nose:** The center between your nose and your upper lip.

6. **Chin point:** The center between your lower lip and your chin.
7. **Beginning of the collarbone:** The point where your inner collarbone meets your breastbone.
8. **Under the arm:** About 4 inches below your armpit, at the side of your body, close to your chest.
9. **Karate chop:** 1.5 inches below your little finger, slightly above your wrist.

Step 5: Rank the intensity of your emotion after finishing this exercise on a scale of 1-10. Repeat this exercise about three to four times. If the ranking is still high, you can repeat the process until the intensity of the emotion goes down.

What I love about tapping, or the Emotional Freedom Technique, is that it is a holistic process that combines mind, body, and heart. Tapping your body while repeating a mantra or an affirmation is healing genius because it serves simultaneously as grounding and soothing; it brings us back to the body; it is mechanical so we are not going down the rumination or overwhelm rabbit hole; and it allows for a full body reframe and re-memorization of the difficult internal experience. It gives a sense of self-control, which automatically initiates the transmutation sequence.

Remember, emotions and trauma are stored in the body and are often read by our operating system as a massive glitch or gobbledygook. It doesn't know what to do with it. We must address the body, move it out of the body with the body. I want to encourage you here: don't worry about it looking weird or it feeling weird to use the body to release these stored globs of unprocessed emotions which create triggers and eruptions. Tools like EFT, the Dynamic Meditation Method, breath work, yoga, and hip releasing are all ways to move emotions out of the body.

Chapter 6

Preventing NPD Through Emotional Intelligence

IN THIS CHAPTER, I explain how emotional intelligence can help us improve our relationship with ourselves, manage overwhelming emotions, and take preventive measures to prevent young children from developing NPD.

If you have children with a narcissist, the last thing you want is for your kids to develop the same personality traits and behavioral patterns. Children learn behaviors from their parents and caregivers. According to MentalHelp.net, around age four months, infants start imitating facial expressions they observe in others ("Emotional and Social Development and Understanding," n.d., para. 2). By the age of six months, babies already start mimicking the emotions and non-verbal cues that they see in others. At around two years old, toddlers begin to experience a wide range of emotions and learn how to regulate and manage their feelings. By age two, they learn how to use their emotions and behaviors to get what they want. Their ability to feel empathy also starts to develop around the age of two.

I don't have any kids myself, but I've met many women who try to hide their pain in front of their children to protect them. They can't bear to see their little ones trying to comfort them while they are crying. These women not only needed to find ways to protect themselves, but they also needed to protect their children. And that's a huge burden to carry. Unfortunately, no matter how hard these women tried to protect their little ones, they were still exposed to some form of abuse. According to Child Welfare Information Gateway, trauma can have significant effects on a child's brain development and behavior ("The Impact of Trauma on Child Brain Development and Behavior," n.d.). Trauma can affect their neurological development, and as a result, they may experience emotional dysregulation and behavioral challenges, which might require a mental health professional to help them process their trauma ("Understanding the Effects of Maltreatment on Brain Development," n.d.).

Grace makes a good point here about childhood experiences of trauma and the need for emotional intelligence. Untreated trauma can be one of the reasons that a child becomes an adult narcissist. If the child's wounds are not met with compassionate space and an attempt to understand "the why" of certain behaviors, the child may begin to self-hate and thus self-avoid. Forms of self-hate and self-avoidance include addictions, compulsive behaviors, self-harm, bullying, manipulation, and narcissism.

At an early stage in childhood, emotional intelligence looks like just naming and hence normalizing their feelings...feelings in general. Note: this requires an emotionally available parent. In homes where there are addictions, neglect, or abuse, feelings tend to be buried, deflected, or projected, because unless there is an exit available, it's too horrific or dangerous to speak to what's happening; therefore, feelings freeze in the body and this becomes part of the agglomeration of PTSD.

If you notice any behavioral concerns, contact a professional to help you do a proper assessment so they can support your child in the best way possible. As a parent, you can also provide your child with the best possible environment to make them feel safe, nurtured, loved, and supported.

Teaching your kids how to develop emotional intelligence is an effective way to help them process their challenging emotions. The term emotional intelligence was explained by Daniel Goleman in the 1990s, where he explained that emotional intelligence can be measured like the intelligence quotient (IQ). He characterized the emotional quotient (EQ) by five skills and qualities that promote mental and emotional well-being. These five skills teach kids how to be self-aware, how to manage their emotions, how to motivate themselves, how to show empathy, and how to develop social skills. According to Goleman (n.d.), research provides support for social-emotional learning (SEL) in education ("Research Supports SEL," para. 5). Some schools have already started running programs to teach emotional intelligence.

Studies have shown that children who were taught emotional intelligence had the following results compared to other students who didn't:

- Anti-social behavior went down by 10%
- Prosocial behavior went up by 10%
- Academic achievement scores went up by 11%

Emotional intelligence begins to develop in early childhood. Children receive and interpret emotional messages through interactions with their parents, teachers, and their peers. These repeated emotional messages and interactions lay the foundation for a child's emotional outlook and capabilities. According to the National Library of Medicine, during the first three or four years of life, our brain grows to about two thirds its full size, and continues to evolve in complexity (Brain development during the preschool years, by Timothy T. Brown and Terry L. Jernigan, NCBI Article PMC351163). Throughout this period, our emotional part of the brain, called the limbic system, starts developing through social interactions with others. Young children do not know how to express themselves or how to handle unpleasant emotions. Which is why they throw tantrums and have outbursts of anger and frustration. If we teach them how to acknowledge and accept what they are feeling, it would be easier for them to manage their emotions and express them appropriately.

To be able to teach our kids about emotional intelligence, first we must develop our own emotional intelligence. Developing your emotional intelligence will benefit you in many ways. It helps you maintain a positive outlook on life and understand yourself at a deeper level. It opens your mind to new possibilities and allows you to manage stress and overcome challenges with a sense of self-empowerment.

I call this the Era of Emotions because the collective consciousness and traditional medicine have caught up with decades of psychology that posits that unprocessed emotions are the root of most—some holistic practitioners would say all—psychological, physical, and mental illnesses. Freud's discovery of the unconscious began when he pinpointed that his client's arm paralysis began to heal when she began speaking (what he coined as "talk therapy") about her childhood abuse.

The last decades saw the focus on the study of the mind via neuroscience, mindfulness practices, perceptual field, and the power of thoughts creating reality. We are now moving into an era where emotional understanding, acceptance, exploration, and regulation is mainstream. The open discussion of trauma and the use of healing modalities such as psychotherapy, breathwork, psychedelics, and meditation has surged and peaked following the Pandemic. Schools, social media, and even celebrities have normalized the discussion of emotions. Healing is a trend and it is a trend that this planet and its humans desperately need and deserve. Grace's book contributes to this vision and mission.

Let's have a look at the main five characteristics of emotional intelligence.

Self-Knowledge

Emotional intelligence starts with self-awareness and self-knowledge. What does it mean to be self-aware? It means that you are aware of your thoughts, feelings and behaviors. Self-awareness allows you to get to know yourself at a deeper level. It means that you are aware of your strengths and weaknesses. Knowing yourself will help you make better choices aligned with your true values.

If you don't know who you really are, you can easily get carried away with life's distractions and end up doing what others want or expect from you, instead of doing what you really want. Self-awareness also helps you make sense of certain emotions and impulsive reactions.

There is no truer statement than this! As I like to say, get a PhD on your self! When we become experts on any subject, we feel confident and powerful in the world. Why not have that subject be you? The more you know yourself the more you feel safe in your own skin, the more you know how to navigate the world and others, and the more you trust to respond to adversity, which is the very definition of resilience. We can do this through self-knowledge and tools. This is why Grace's book is so powerful because she invites the reader to know themselves and also provides exercises and tools. As best-selling author and healing practitioner, Joe Dispenza says, "It's not enough to know. We must know how."

When I started doing inner reflection, I started questioning what I thought was real and truthful, why I did certain things, and why I made certain decisions. This step is key to change and transformation. As you shed light on your unconscious beliefs about yourself and the world around you, you realize what you need to do to change the direction of your life. Self-knowledge is power!

I'd like to add why self-knowledge and the willingness to self-explore is a key distinction between the wounded Empath or the victim, and the narcissist. We see that the wounded Empath or victim may have the exact same childhood trajectory as the narcissist: trauma, abuse, neglect, feelings of profound inferiority, existential emptiness, abandonment fear, and more often than not, an indulgent focus on their own suffering.

Where the wounded Empath or victim parts ways with the narcissist and what makes them different from the narcissist, is their willingness to self-reflect! The narcissist will not turn inward but will rather blame everyone and everything else for their woes. The victim or the wounded Empath is willing to ask themselves deeper questions about their own behavior. This can be to their detriment if engaged with a blaming narcissist, but it can also be the very key to their healing, as we see here in Grace's story. Grace was willing to study the situation, learn about the dynamics, and self-reflect about her own involvement. This characteristic—an emotionally intelligent one—opened up the portal to her healing and spiritual journey.

Teaching children to pay attention to what they're feeling and asking them to express themselves with words helps them build self-awareness. Building self-awareness helps them deal with overwhelming emotions and control impulsive reactions. Emotional literacy can also reduce bullying at school. According to the University of Washington (2006), exposure to violence in the home is linked to increased rates of childhood bullying ("Violence in the Home Leads to Higher Rates of Childhood Bullying," para. 1). With self-awareness, children learn how to understand themselves at a deeper level and communicate their emotions in a healthy way.

Self-Control

Have you ever had an argument and said some hurtful things which you regretted later? Or perhaps you had an outburst of anger, and you didn't know how to control it? Learning how to observe our emotions without trying to repress them, and without acting out on the impulses, enables us to express our emotions in a healthy way which doesn't involve harming others. So, what does self-control look like? It doesn't mean that you don't allow yourself to feel your emotions. It means that you are being conscious and mindful, even during challenging emotions and impulses like anger, or rage. As you invite awareness when you feel the emotional impulse arising within you, you can quickly analyze how you can express and release this emotion without harming others or yourself. Self-control gives you power as you learn how to respond consciously to situations instead of acting on autopilot.

Teaching kids how to be mindful and identify what sensations they are feeling in their body can help them express their emotions differently. Just like any other skill, self-control can be taught. This skill will be extremely useful later on in their adult life as they continue to face challenging situations which might trigger unpleasant emotions. Learning how to process different emotions can help children navigate through life's challenges and build sustainable relationships.

Personal Motivation for Self-Growth

What motivates you as an individual? Do you know what you need to do to get yourself motivated when you feel like you're stuck in a rut? Knowing what motivates us helps us feel alive, energized, joyful, and with a healthy appetite for life. The benefits of motivation are reflected in our lives as we become more adaptable to change, learn new behaviors and skills, set goals, raise children, and feel engaged in our own lives.

When we are depleted of motivation, we find ourselves feeling apathetic, and it negatively impacts our overall well-being. And when we are faced with challenging situations, we feel powerless against them.

Knowing what motivates you encourages you to find the strength within you and motivate yourself to keep going and push through. It's easier to stay hopeful and positive minded when you are motivated. Otherwise, you'll fall into the trap of looking at the glass half empty and start focusing on the negative things in life. Motivation promotes self-growth and equips you with the momentum and power that you need in order to continue growing and learning.

If we teach our kids at a young age how to be curious and find out what motivates them, it will be easier for them to maintain good mental health despite the difficulties they might be facing at home. Motivation empowers them to overcome difficult situations which they might come across. It helps them grow and see the positive things in life. Through my experiences I've learned that we cannot control anything that happens outside of us. The only power we have is over ourselves. This realization helped me stay motivated as I understood that I always had a choice. No matter what was happening around me, I could choose to either surrender and be defeated, or find my inner strength to continue growing, learning, and moving forward.

Empathy

Since I was a kid, I always remember my mum telling me to be kind to others, to help others, and to treat everyone with respect. When other kids in school were mean to their peers, I couldn't understand why and how they could be so hurtful with their words and behaviors. Later on, I discovered that we are not born with empathy, it's a skill that needs to be learned. And just like any other skill, like learning a language or riding a bike, the earlier you start developing it in life, the better.

An empathic person is considerate of other people's feelings as they can feel and understand what another person is going through. Teaching kids at a young age to empathize with each other helps them understand different views and perceptions. As a result, they are less likely to participate in fights and more likely to understand different points of views without judgment. People with a high level of empathy are generally more compassionate and hold value in uplifting others. They treat everyone with respect and are able to build strong connections with others.

Empathy is the core to safe and sound relationships; in fact, it is the main social skill for connecting with others, known or unknown. I call this the "I am you and you are me" principle. When you deeply and fearlessly know yourself, including your most difficult, vulnerable, and unattractive parts, and have compassion for yourself, you can extend this grace to others. When we understand that we all have human emotions and human responses to life, we can have empathy for the same in others.

Neuroscientifically, we have a particular set of neurons called "mirror neurons." The way these work is that when we gaze upon another and we see what they are doing, we will imitate or respond to that behavior. I find that knowing ourselves profoundly allows for the same type of psychological function; we know and accept others because we know and accept ourselves. I am you and you are me, or, when I teach this phrase: "When I deeply know me, I can get you."

Social Skills

Whether we like it or not, we are social beings and the quality of our life strongly depends on the quality of our relationships. Self-confidence and good communication skills help us excel in social settings. A person that is highly emotionally intelligent with good social skills is able to integrate with others efficiently without feeling the need to be superior. Narcissists might come across as having good social skills, but due to their fragile egos, the need to feel superior, and disregard of other people's feelings, they are not able to build intimate and authentic relationships. They are always on the lookout for something they can benefit from through their relationships with others.

If our children learn how to develop good social skills, they are less likely to feel a lack of sense of belonging. Connecting with others and a sense of belonging is important for people to feel whole and loved. It makes us feel like we are part of something bigger. That's why community work is so rewarding and fulfilling.

Teaching emotional literacy is important for children to develop self-confidence and a healthy self-esteem.

I would add to this section that emotional literacy is available to adults as well, no matter what they experienced in the past. One of my specialties is teaching people with ADHD, C-PTSD, General Anxiety Disorder, and Empaths how to know, regulate, and calibrate their emotions. I compiled my best spiritual, meditational, clinical, and psychological principles, tools, and processes to create the Dynamic Meditation Method where people feel like they have both the knowledge and the know-how to handle their internal experience in real time and in the long run. Ultimately, the Dynamic Meditation Method is a source of self-esteem through emotional prowess, and it all starts with the simple, willing step of going inside to self-discover.

It acts like an internal moral and navigating compass. The basic principle that children must learn is that it's okay to feel and experience unpleasant emotions, however, there's a way of dealing with them and expressing them. When this is modeled for them, they learn that acting out is not okay. Unfortunately, many children are taught the opposite, and instead of teaching them to accept and deal with their emotions, they learn that they need to repress their emotions, and be the best in everything in our competitive society.

There are signs and indications that show if a child is prone to developing NPD. If you notice these warning signs in teenagers, there's an indicating risk of developing narcissism:

- Engaging in persistent bullying
- Needing to win no matter who is hurt
- Persistent lying to benefit oneself
- Deflecting accountability to wrongdoing
- Grandiose sense of self-worth
- Extremely selfish and preoccupied with getting own needs met over other people's needs
- Feeling entitled to special treatment
- Aggressive reactions to criticism
- Blaming others for bad outcomes

There are several factors that could result in developing NPD like genetic predisposition, personality traits, environmental conditions, and social interactions. There's no guaranteed way to prevent NPD, however, by collectively taking certain measures, we can prevent children from developing severe symptoms of this mental health issue. We can also prevent victims from falling prey to their manipulative games by raising awareness, and by teaching people how to recognize the signs and symptoms of NPD. Societal interventions like prevention of child abuse, domestic violence, and substance abuse can also help decrease mental health problems, like narcissistic personality disorder.

If you observe these behavioral traits in your child, you can save your family and society from potential harm by teaching them emotional literacy. It's also highly recommended to speak to a professional therapist to provide the best treatment as deemed appropriate. Teaching and helping children cultivate emotional intelligence can save our communities on a global level from a lot of unnecessary harm. Together we can contribute to creating a better world, a global community ruled by love, kindness and compassion.

INSIGHTFUL LESSON: We cannot control anything that happens outside of us. The only power we have is over ourselves.

Simple Exercises to Increase Emotional Intelligence

#1. Take some quiet time for yourself. Reflect on what kind of events trigger your emotions. Identify what emotions are triggered. What do you believe about yourself for these emotions to be triggered?

#2. Have conscious conversations with yourself. Ask yourself, *"How am I feeling today?" "Why do I feel this way?"* Start noticing how you speak to yourself. Sometimes, we don't realize how mean we can be to ourselves. If you notice that you are being harsh on yourself, ask yourself whether you would speak to a dear friend that way. Change your self-sabotage talk and start talking to yourself with kindness and compassion.

#3. Observe what kind of behaviors and choices are linked to particular thoughts and emotions. For example:

INTERCONNECTION OF THOUGHTS, FEELINGS, AND BEHAVIORS

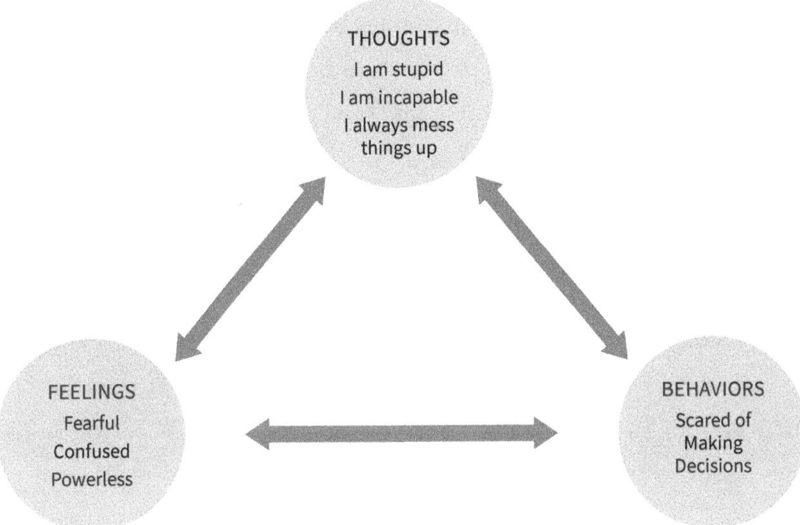

#4. Rephrase these thoughts into supportive thoughts that empower you. For example:

I can take care of myself (*thought*) → **Empowered (*feeling*)** → **Making an important decision (*behavior*)**

#5. When you get into an argument with the narcissist and you get triggered, invite awareness and take a three second pause before you reply or act. Ask yourself whether it's wise to act with impulsivity, or whether it would be more beneficial to reply with silence. It's highly likely that if you allow yourself to get heated up in the argument, you will end up feeling frustrated, angry and depleted of energy. Deciding not to participate in pointless arguments helps you conserve your energy and protect yourself from negative energy.

Identifying Your Emotions in Your Body

Step 1: Find yourself a quiet space and make sure you won't be disturbed. Sit down on a chair making sure that your back is straight and supported, with your feet grounded on the floor. You can also choose to lay down if this feels more comfortable for you.

Step 2: Take three deep mindful breaths as you bring your attention to the present moment.

Step 3: Notice whether you have any tension in different parts of your body. Do your muscles feel tense? Or perhaps you feel anxiety in your chest or your stomach? Does your jaw feel tight or perhaps you notice any tension around your forehead or the crown of your head?

Step 4: Continue to breathe deeply as you focus your attention on different parts of your body. Notice if any sensations come up and just observe them without judgment.

Step 5: Listen to your body and ask yourself what you need to do to release this emotion. Your body carries universal intelligence and it will guide you. Don't try to control what comes next, just listen gently and trust your body.

Step 6: You might feel the need to make some gestures with your hand or move your body in a particular way. You might feel the need to cry out loud. Trust yourself, listen to your body and give it what it needs. These emotions are not for you to hold on to.

Step 7: Emotions are energy in motion. If you keep them trapped in your body they can cause physical discomfort and inflammation. Wrap your arms around yourself and support yourself with love.

What I can add here is not an exercise but a foundational principle that I teach in Dynamic. It is the "I am you and you are me" principle." I find that it defines emotional intelligence from an unusual, thorough, and visceral angle. The "I am you and you are me" principle posits that we are one and the same: whether it be through the lens of quantum physics in that we are all entangled at a subatomic level; whether it be anthropologically and we all come from the same human species; or whether it be mechanically, that we all have the same operating system (emotions) that is designed to help us distinguish our uniqueness as well as join us in our sameness.

The process of deeply exploring, understanding, and transmuting our feelings allows us to identify feelings like shame, guilt, fear, disgust, lust, glee (believe it or not, glee is a feeling that is quite repressed in adults), and so on. Once we have truly "crawled" our way through these emotional tunnels, de-shame, and accept them, we are not only able to identify them in another, we are more powerfully able to connect with another. We can understand another's emotional reactions and responses even when we don't share the same story. What we share are the same emotional touchpoints.

The miracle of 12-step programs or psychotherapy groups is the experience of having people from all walks of life, most often very divergent walks of life, come together in a circle of emotional understanding and acceptance. The emotions themselves are the common human language, which is why we can cry or laugh when witnessing movie scenes, images, or memes from other cultures. Emotional intelligence is thus the ability to recognize and understand another's emotional world through the process of having explored one's own. There are many processes, groups, modalities, and tools such as the ones Grace is providing, that assist on this arduous internal journey of deeply experiencing our feelings. It is an extra bonus to know that beyond healing and trauma rising, we emerge

Chapter 7

Can NPD Be Cured?

WHEN I WAS STILL in the relationship, I was hopeful that one day he would realize how unjust he was being with me. There were times when I had built up the courage to leave, yet the false hope of him improving held me stuck in the relationship. He used to charm his way back into my life and fill my head with false promises. I fell for his tricks every time. There were days where we sat at our kitchen table, and we talked for hours about his behaviors and his personality disorder. He used to tell me that he's aware of what's happening and that he's being exploitative of me.

But for him, using others for his own needs and hidden motives was not immoral. He felt entitled to have that right over others. To justify his behavior, he told me that I should have been smart enough to realize what was happening a long time ago. And since I "wasn't smart enough" to realize it by myself, he said that I deserved to be treated that way.

These kinds of conversations never got me anywhere. The following day I used to confront him to hold him accountable, but he used to deny our conversations. As you can imagine, I used to feel outraged. The more this happened, the more I realized that he was just wasting my precious time. To ensure that I had tried everything in my power to try and make him change, I went to seek guidance from a psychologist. I explained to her everything that was happening between us and how he was treating me, and she informed me that he should speak to her urgently.

Of course, he refused to do so, and he pointed out to me that he felt proud for being that way as it meant that he was above standard and better than others. It hurt my brain to hear him speak in such a way. The psychologist informed me that personality traits of narcissistic personality disorder are extremely difficult to change. One of the most challenging aspects for them is admitting that something is not right with them. It is highly unlikely that an individual with a fully blown narcissistic personality disorder will seek therapy. If they do, it's either because they have been forced by someone close to them, or because they hit rock bottom due to their self-destructive behaviors.

Even when they hit rock bottom, psychotherapy becomes merely another source of supply. Narcissists are willing to either pay extensively for psychotherapy or play the victim to maintain the therapist as a source of supply. In my experience with NPD cases, the relational sequence is the same. First, they are quite seductive in their storytelling, they are entertaining and appear vulnerable at first, and they either speak very highly of themselves or lowly, as they gauge what will work best for them. Second, they begin to establish dominance with the therapist, whether it be by asking personal questions, alluding to something they know about you, and possibly using it against you.

An example for me was a client who knew that my son was biracial and let me know, and in sessions would demean that particular race while claiming that my son was the exception. Sessions do not serve the purpose of self-growth but rather are psychologically masturbatory; the NPD client uses the therapist and the session to only talk about themselves without and is not interested in true feedback or change. It's important to note that they will charm, beg, or pay more when they feel that the therapist will terminate with them.

I no longer see NPD clients because it requires an extreme amount of fortitude and wherewithal to see past the mirage and seductive storytelling. They can also make you feel extremely needed, and if the therapist is inexperienced or has a history of unprocessed narcissistic wounding, they can get trapped in a codependent cycle. My suggestion for therapists working with NPD clients is the standard suggestion for any therapist who works with AXIS II/personality disorders: have consistent collegial support and expertise in the topic is non-negotiable.

Even if they agree to seek therapy, it may take several years before you start seeing a sign of improvement. Until they see some kind of results, they might begin to see therapy as a waste of time and be tempted to quit. Moreover, having to discuss their emotions and challenging questions with their therapist can be extremely difficult and uncomfortable for them. Their brain has been programmed in a way to protect itself from seeing who they really have become. Most narcissists don't want to appear as bad people and give great importance to their reputation and social status. So even if they start doing therapy, according to the information provided on Psych Central, narcissistic personality disorder is a lifelong mental health disorder, and there is no cure for it ("Narcissism Cure," n.d.).

If you're stuck in a relationship with a narcissist, or you are finding it hard to get over one, it might be because you are still hoping that things could be better between you. When you really understand how deeply entwined these personality traits are in their psyche, you start accepting the fact that things cannot get any better. Accepting that you can't do anything to improve the situation will help you let go of the need to "be" better and fix things. At some point, you decided that this was your problem to fix. Why would you want to hold on to something that is causing you so much pain and suffering? What makes life so difficult without this person?

Later on in this book, I will share with you how I learned to shift my focus on myself so I could heal all that needed to be healed. Once I learned how to love myself and set boundaries, I felt whole and complete without needing anyone to make me feel worthy. I was able to shift my perception from being a victim, to being a warrior who turned her pain into purpose.

Checking In with Yourself

When you're struggling to make a decision, do this exercise to seek guidance through your *internal guidance system*:

Step 1: Mind Perception (Analytical, Keep Us Safe, Limited)

Close your eyes. Take three deep, mindful breaths. Put your hand on your head. Ask yourself a question about a problem you are having and perceive the problem from your mind. Ask yourself, what can I do about it? Go through different perceptions and write them down.

Step 2: Gut Feeling (Intuition)

Close your eyes. Take three deep, mindful breaths. Place your hand on your stomach. Consider the problem from your gut and see what your instinct tells you. How else can you perceive this and resolve this? Write them down.

Step 3: Heart (Truth, Knowing, Vulnerability, Courage)

Close your eyes. Take three deep, mindful breaths. Place your hand on your heart.

Perceive the situation from your heart. What are some other ways you can deal with this in your life? What do you need to learn, heal, do or understand to resolve this? Write them down.

When struggling to make a decision, when you're ping-ponging back and forth, or when you're in "should I stay or should I go" mode, as the Clash song says, I use a Dynamic Exercise called "Attachments and Aversions." I learned the attachments and aversions exercise through Lester Levinson' s work, a physicist whose self-healing, energetic processes I use as core tools in the Dynamic Meditation Method.

The exercise sounds like a pros and cons list, but it is not. It is actually a very efficient and powerful way to "pop" the unconscious and reach the deeper layers of why the decision is so difficult and confusing. The exercise is quite mechanical and must be done all the way through so that it sifts through the confusion and lands on the most aligned answer. Have a picture that as you do the process, you are peeling away the layers that are burying the answer.

This exercise can often feel tedious, and the answer may be revealed a few hours or days later but know that it works like a charm and is an actual written meditation in that it's cleaning up the confusion clutter that is usually paralyzing. Remember that the writing part is the grounding aspect in the swirl of indecision.

At the top of a sheet of paper, write the title of your indecision, for example, "Being Alone." Underneath the title, make two columns and above each column write "Advantage" and "Disadvantage" respectively. Number each column from 1-8 lines. Ask, "What is the advantage of being alone?" Have the answer pop—no long paragraphs or analysis—just pop the unconscious. Write the quick answer and then ask, "Is this about wanting safety, control, or approval?" These are the three survival programs that unconsciously run in all humans. Choose one or all three survival programs. Quickly move to the second column and ask, "What is the disadvantage of being alone?" Pop and answer and then ask which survival program it triggers. It is imperative that you keep asking those same questions over and over until you have completed the eight on each.

Part III

Why Are We Attracted to Narcissists?

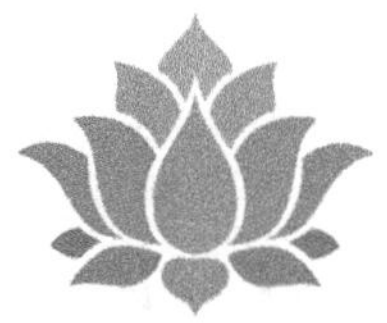

LET'S FACE IT, NARCISSISTS come off as charming, confident, successful, and above standard. Everyone can fall for their act and love-bombing, even successful and self-confident men and women so don't be too hard on yourself. There's a difference between being tricked and manipulated into a narcissistic relationship, or always finding yourself in abusive relationships. If you're anything like me, I felt like I was a magnet to narcissists. I was surrounded by narcissists at different workplaces, family members, friends, and romantic relationships. Was it just me or was there something behind the scenes going on which I seemed to be missing?

What a good and worthwhile question! If we place this question in the addictive framework, the rephrasing is "What is the meaning of insanity? Doing the same thing over and over and expecting different results." We must change if we want change. Unless the childhood wound is healed, the adult child of an alcoholic will always attract the alcoholic in the room, and they will "serendipitously" find each other.

From a spiritual perspective, our external landscape will be a reflection of our internal landscape. In Karmic terms, what lesson kept reappearing for it to be solved and upleveled. A good question for Grace here was, what relational dynamic was established in childhood that is repeating itself? What are the variables, for example: people pleasing or fawning as a defense mechanism which surely attracts more dominant types; savior tendencies if someone appears in need; giving-to-get tendencies which can stem from having to give to the caregiver in order to feel loved or feel parented; and another amongst many, is the attraction to intensity, possibly even dramatic intensity, if the child was brought up in an explosive home or with intermittent parenting.

Understanding these relational formulas inside oneself can assist in breaking the pattern by shifting the variables.

After my breakup, I had developed a strong radar for narcissists. So, by then I could tell that these people were narcissistic, and I felt like I needed to protect myself from them. I had to fight my instinct and resist this intense energetic field that was attracting more narcissists into my reality. The attraction was too intense, and I found myself repeating the same mistakes and getting involved with more narcissistic romantic partners. I felt like a magnetic pull towards these men. It was like an invisible force that was stronger than me was drawing me towards them. Being aware of these dynamics between me and narcissists got me curious. Why did they feel so irresistible and why was I especially attracted to these kinds of men?

You know how they say opposites attract, the law of polarity described perfectly how I felt when I was approached by these people. The law of polarity describes the principle of two opposite poles, that everything in the universe has its opposite. Like north and south poles, negative and positive on a battery, light and darkness, masculine and feminine, etc. My kind of personality fitted perfectly with a narcissist thanks to my dysfunctional behavioral habits and inner core beliefs. I could tell that these narcissistic men were experiencing the same tension around me. It's as if we were predestined to cross each other's paths. Some people describe this as a *"karmic relationship."*

This description made perfect sense to me and helped me realize that I needed to break this karmic relationship to break free from the toxic cycle. By no means am I saying that this is your karma and that you deserve to pay your karma in the currency of suffering and abuse. And this shouldn't be interpreted as a justifiable reason for staying in an abusive relationship. It's actually the complete opposite. The karmic relationship happens with one objective: *"To point you into the direction of the universal Truth, to learn what you still need to learn to remember who you are and return to love."* After doing a great deal of inner work and introspection, I realized that life was trying to teach me a lesson. Until

I became aware of what was happening, I kept finding myself attracted to the same type of person over and over again, experiencing the same heartache. Once I cracked the code, I realized that I needed to work on the relationship with myself to start making different choices.

Right on, Grace. The wound becomes a gift we can apply to the lesson learned. I always say, "Don't feel it for free," since some of the feelings are so intense and painful. The journey must be worth the alchemized gold we have at the end: the higher, more evolved version of oneself.

Through meditation and other spiritual practices, I was able to shift my perception and view what was happening to me from a different perspective. Instead of perceiving myself as a helpless victim, I moved away from self-pity and started perceiving myself as an active participant in my life journey. I started questioning what kind of choices I had made that got me into this kind of relationship. It took me years to heal, learn, and break the cycle. From then onwards, I started holding myself accountable for my decisions and realized that I was responsible for my mistakes and my own happiness. This realization helped me to stop seeking happiness outside of me and trying to make myself feel whole through the validation of other people.

Holding herself accountable and realizing that happiness was her responsibility upleveled Grace into a sovereign human with agency. By becoming a decision-maker of her own fortune, per se, she would automatically begin to repel the narcissist because he can no longer "plug in" to her low self-esteem and willingness to do anything to feel seen. Grace moved from questioning herself to questioning behaviors outside of her that no longer suited her well-being. The narcissist does not like to have motives or behaviors questioned. This is an enormous and profound shift.

If you keep finding yourself being attracted to narcissists, you might wonder why you keep attracting them into your life. With self-reflection and by discovering what beliefs you hold about yourself, you can identify why you keep attracting narcissists and why you choose to stay in abusive relationships.

Childhood wounds such as abuse, neglect, fear of abandonment, and anxious or disorganized attachment styles come into play here. We repeat what we grew up with, we seek what we didn't get, and we will pay very high prices to fulfill caregiving needs that we did not receive as children.

Also worth addressing is the age-old question that outside people wonder and often ask directly: "Why did you stay? Why didn't you leave if it was that bad?"

Not only can learned helplessness be emphasized enough—the constant abusive conditioning that belittles the human to believing that they are nothing without the narcissist—but the fact that the narcissist is an expert at isolating the victim to such an extent that the victim feels like they have no place to go. All allies have been rejected or made to be enemies. Most outside people, if whole in their own right, will not want to be around the narcissist because they see or sense their destructive nature.

To compound the matter of staying with the narcissist, is the erosion of truth; the victim can no longer identify what is true anymore because their own truth has been repetitively questioned and they have been punished or demeaned for even having an opinion on truth. The rabbit hole of self-doubt and self-hate is like a tomb the victim is buried under, and it impedes any urge to leave. The question "why didn't you leave?" only adds to the despairing shame that is characteristic of that relationship.

In this chapter, I talk about the main elements which are present in those who end up victims to narcissistic abuse. Most often, it's a mix of all these elements and characteristics in our personality that match us up with narcissistic people. These characteristics make us the perfect prey for narcissists. At the end of each chapter, you will find exercises and easy steps which you can follow to change these unhealthy behavioral habits and transform into a better version of yourself. This will help you heal your emotional wounds and learn how to protect yourself from other narcissists which you might come across in your life.

- **INSIGHTFUL LESSON:** A karmic relationship happens to point us to the direction of the universal truth so we can remember who we really are and return to love.

Chapter 8

Blurred Boundaries

WHAT ARE BOUNDARIES? WHAT'S the difference between blurred boundaries and solid boundaries? Before going through all of this, I had no idea what boundaries were. No one had ever taught me how to set boundaries or explained to me why it's important to establish solid boundaries.

What does having blurred boundaries sound like?

- Saying yes when you really wanted to say no.
- Agreeing to help others even when it's inconvenient for you.
- Sacrificing your own needs to please others.
- Feeling guilty when saying no to others.
- Allowing people to walk over you.
- Let others push their beliefs on you.
- Struggling to be assertive.
- Being scared to voice your own opinion.
- Feeling guilty when others are upset around you.
- Letting others make decisions for you.

Struggling to set and hold boundaries is a core issue in narcissistic relationships. If you're a people pleaser and find it difficult to say no to people, it means that you have issues with setting boundaries. People with blurred boundaries find it difficult to assert their needs and to express themselves, so they end up accepting just about anything to avoid having conflict. Setting boundaries might trigger feelings of guilt where you end up feeling responsible for other people's emotions.

Setting boundaries can also trigger intense abandonment fears. This is so key. As a child, if a caregiver was intermittent, present then absent, or directly threatened to leave, the child will grow up with a terrified internal experience of being left alone. Defenses for this can look like being the extremely "good" child, who doesn't ask for anything, doesn't fret or fuss, and certainly who doesn't say no to anything that the adult may want in order to not be abandoned.

Remember, neglect and abandonment for a small one literally threatens their core sense of survival. They thus develop survival skills that include being "very good," being the "best little helper," and never, ever putting their needs first, and possibly never even knowing their needs.

Having difficulty maintaining solid boundaries can be a result of different environmental experiences in your childhood. For example, people who were brought up in an enmeshed family usually have unclear personal boundaries, which are not clearly defined.

An important point about boundaries and enmeshment is that the fabric of some cultures and ethnicities is woven with enmeshment. Boundaries may be seen as disrespectful, rejecting, arrogant, or superior. Some cultures base their relationships with their children entirely on co-dependence, and an expectation that the children live for the parents. Despite being adults who may be married, have their own children, or are independent.

As a Latina psychotherapist, I not only know this in my own skin and upbringing and had to work through it, but I have to identify and understand cultural norms with which my clients were raised. The therapeutic work of individuation—a term coined by Carl Jung to describe a human's self-actualization journey towards the authentic self, separate from their parents and upbringing, but psychologically mature enough to remain connected—must be examined within a cultural context.

So, it becomes difficult for family members to develop a healthy level of autonomy and independence. When these individuals interact with other people outside their family, they find it difficult to maintain solid boundaries, as they never really learned how to do it.

Struggling to set solid boundaries could also be the result of receiving bad reactions from your caregivers when trying to assert yourself at home. Through your past life experiences you've learned that setting boundaries causes conflict and upsets others. It's an indirect message telling you that your voice and opinion do not matter. If you're used to being ignored when you try to set boundaries, it means that you have been conditioned that way and it becomes a subconscious world map which you unknowingly use to navigate through life.

The inability to set solid boundaries makes you an ideal candidate for a narcissist. Narcissists don't respect boundaries. They start testing you from the very beginning of the relationship to see how much they are able to get away with. What you allow to happen will continue happening! Every time you accept and justify their behavior, you indirectly tell the narcissist that your boundaries can be pushed, and that you can be manipulated to submit to whatever he or she wants.

As sadistic as this sounds, what Grace highlights here is true. The narcissist is strategically identifying what your perimeters and parameters are. In the honeymoon stage, the stage where you may feel most "seen and known," is very likely because they are detailing you in every way and measuring what works, what gets your attention, and most importantly, what will get them the most supply. For some, it's love bombing, for others it's acting like they need saving, being steadfastly present, and so on. They will start pushing the boundaries—financial, physical, and emotional—to see how far the victim will go.

Once they have made that assessment, all bets are off and the boundaries will be pushed even further and likely annihilated. Remember, for most people with a kind heart, children, or a neglected human, it seems normal to respond caringly to someone's needs or request for help. The issue is when it becomes emotional molestation, i.e., the use of the kind or neglected heart, to self-serve and abuse.

At first, you might not realize that the narcissist is pushing your boundaries. But at some point in your life, you look at your relationship and realize how unhappy you are. And that is what happens when you are not living aligned with your true values. You realize that you've accepted much more than you were at first willing to accept. When you're in a relationship with a narcissist, it's so easy to get stuck in the loop of justification. You don't realize how much of yourself you've given up hanging onto the illusionary ending of you two being happy together. Ignoring your values and principles is not sustainable long term, it leads to extreme amounts of stress, suffering, and soul depletion.

Throughout our relationship, I gave him countless ultimatums and conditions. I refused to see that I had no control over him or the relationship whatsoever. Towards the end of our relationship, I decided to make a list of the pros and cons of the relationship. I also listed my most important values that I wanted to live with to see whether these values were present in our relationship.

I love highlighting Grace's (and my clients') moments of self-love and what I see as their inner being's acts of r-evolution. Moments such as detailing her values and measuring them against the actual relationship was her higher self, her soul, her inner being reminding her of who she was. Yes! And this became an actual tool that paved the way for liberation.

MY VALUES	MY RELATIONSHIP
Loyalty	He was not loyal to anyone, including family members, friends and previous romantic partners. He bad-mouthed everyone and talked behind other people's backs, even against his own best friends.
Faithfulness	He was only faithful to himself. He was not a man of his word as he constantly made false promises.
Trust	He broke my trust from the beginning of the relationship by flirting with other girls. Other girls were always coming between us in our relationship.
Honesty	He was constantly lying about everything. He denied that he was lying even when caught red handed. He had hidden motives and wasn't honest about his intentions and feelings for me.
Integrity	He had no sense of moral values or principles. He made his own rules which only benefited him and he bent his rules whenever it suited him.

MY VALUES	MY RELATIONSHIP
Respect	He told me multiple times that I hadn't earned his respect yet because I hadn't proven myself. He disrespected me and made fun of me in front of other people. He disrespected my needs, my boundaries, my emotions, my family and my friends. He disrespected his family members and friends whenever he felt like it.
Security	He didn't make me feel safe. He made me feel fearful, anxious and stressed, always on edge. He threatened me with words to manipulate me into doing whatever he wanted.
Kindness	He was mean with his words and often talked badly about everyone. He only did acts of kindness with a hidden motive, whenever it benefited him.
Compassion	He didn't feel compassion for people because he believed that they get what they deserve.
Empathy	He was not able to empathize with me. He was not able to empathize with others. He faked empathy in different social contexts when it was good for his reputation.

This is a beautiful tool for any relationship and a defining moment of individuation. We are often not given this roadmap, these relational instructions to apply when we begin to partner with others, even co-workers. This era, epitomized by this book, marks an enormous step in human evolution, as we no longer have to be emotionally spastic human beings, disempowered by not knowing ourselves; we rather are deep diving into the PhD of our own, beautiful selves.

As you can see, he was the complete opposite of what I was looking for in a relationship. Yet somehow, this wasn't clear to me before. I hadn't realized that I was holding on to a person who was so different from what I actually wanted. And that's why knowing who you really are and what you want out of life is so important. It needs to be crystal clear in your head so you know who is aligned with your values and who isn't. Maintaining solid boundaries means that when you come across a person who is not aligned with your values, you accept that you are not compatible and move on. You don't try to bend over backwards and force things into a certain direction.

Grace makes such a great point here about accepting incompatibilities. It is understandable if knowing your needs, wants, and values takes a while on the relationship journey, and embedded in Grace's point is the very subtle but profound principle that knowing yourself via your unique and personal preferences automatically repels what is not for you (because it can't "plug in") or helps you walk away when you are misaligned.

After I spent some time reflecting on this list, it became clear to me what a mess I was in. I realized that I had to go within myself and start learning how to set solid boundaries and maintain them. I hadn't built up the courage to break up with him yet, but I knew I had to start from somewhere. The shift in my perception towards the meaning of the term *"boundaries"* was a game changer for me. Prior to this shift in perception, for me, boundaries meant pushing someone I loved away from me. It meant feeling guilty for asserting my needs and for communicating my feelings.

I feel that Grace's journey of self-understanding provides us with hope. Even when relationships are dysfunctional and destructive, through our internal work, we can use them for reflection and a redesign, if you will, of who we are and who we want to be. I hold with conviction that our wounds—even our deepest ones—can alchemize into our greatest life gifts. I call this Trauma Rising. Grace and I are aligned in this belief as is demonstrated through the title of this book.

This list helped me realize that having boundaries is a way of honoring my values and choosing to live in alignment with my principles. I understood that if I wanted to be happy in life, I needed to respect my values and morals. Otherwise, I was going to keep finding myself in a continuous internal conflict between the life I am living, and who I really am.

Try out the exercise to understand yourself at a deeper level and see what values are important to you. In the first column, list the most important values and principles you wish to live in alignment with. In the second column, write down how your partner behaves in accordance with your values and principles.

Self-Reflective Exercise: My Important Values

This exercise will help you have a clear idea of what is important for you. If your choices are not aligned with your values, you are not living according to your truth. If you want to build healthy, loving relationships, your relationship needs to have these values and principles respected.

INSIGHTFUL LESSON: Setting boundaries is not selfish. Boundaries are like a protective shield to protect you from all that is not good for you.

Building Boundaries Around Your Needs & Values

Step 1: Take some time to reflect on your needs and values. Write them down. (Ex: need for intimate connection, value honesty).

Step 2: Notice how you feel when your needs and values aren't respected. Write down your feelings. (Ex: need for intimate connection → disrespected → feel lonely and rejected).

Step 3: Think of what you would like from your ideal partner to respect your needs and values. Write it down. (Ex: need for intimate connection → build an authentic intimate relationship based on unconditional love and support).

Step 4: Reflect on what choices you need to make to respect your values, needs, and boundaries in relationships. Write them down. (Ex: need for intimate connection → when someone is emotionally unavailable or unable to build an authentic relationship → I choose to leave the relationship because I respect and honor my needs for my own good)

Easy-to-Follow Steps to Set Boundaries

Step 1: Take some time to reflect on what kind of situations make you feel triggered.

Step 2: Identify and write down your emotions.

Step 3: See if you notice any bodily sensations. Where do you feel this emotion in your body?

Step 4: Ask yourself: 'Why am I feeling this way?'

Step 5: Reflect on what you would like to say and how you can say it. Write it down. (Ex: Need for space → "I need some quiet time by myself to unwind.")

Step 6: Write down what might happen if you don't communicate your needs. How would your life be impacted in the short term?

Now, fast forward five years. Imagine yourself still not setting boundaries. How do you feel? How has this affected your emotional and mental well-being? Your relationships? Your self-worth?

Step 7: Write down what might happen if you do communicate your needs. How would your life be impacted in the short term?

Now, fast forward five years. Imagine yourself confidently setting boundaries and honoring your needs. How do you feel? How has this improved your emotional and mental well-being? Your relationships? Your self-worth?

Chapter 9

Codependency

BEFORE DISCOVERING WHAT CODEPENDENCY was, I thought that my choices and behaviors were just me being me. Since I was a kid, I have always remembered having this need to help and save others. If someone in the room or in my social group was feeling sad or distressed, I felt like I was responsible for their feelings, and I went out of my way to help them feel better.

Grace is an Empath, and I capitalize this word because I use it as a proper noun. Empaths lead their life via their kind heart and tend to see the good in others, even when they have been deeply wounded. The Empath is not just "empathic"; the Empath's keen ability to relate to what others feel goes beyond empathy to actually feeling what others are feeling and experiencing in their own body. It's a sensorimotor telepathy of sorts. Empaths connect with others—even strangers—on a deep level that goes beyond logic and words, and have an uncanny ability to read people and energies in a room with great precision.

However, unless the Empath is taught, validated, or trained about their capacities, they may be either dismissed or bullied into questioning and suppressing what they are energetically reading and dismissing it themselves. This is the danger when in a relationship with a Narcissist. Not only will the narcissist gaslight the Empath, but the Empath will also invalidate themselves, stemming from early childhood experiences.

Empaths are often the saviors, fixers, problem-solvers with their families, friends, and love relationships because they are hard-wired for maintaining harmony, and in order to feel harmony (in their own bodies), they feel compelled to solve most issues externally. Over time, this savior/solver identity becomes a way they are loved and thus automatically attracts people and situations (even workplaces) that require those skills. The unhealed Empath is an easy mark for the narcissist because they are a near limitless source of supply, as they will go on overdrive to harmonize the environment, and because they see and want the good from the narcissist.

I approach the relationship with the narcissist from the Empath point of view. My expertise on the topic covers what it means to be an Empath, who they are when they are wounded, why they so perfectly fit with a narcissist when they haven't self-healed, and how they can begin their journey to self-healing, empowerment, and even leadership.

World-renowned psychiatrist and psychoanalyst Carl Jung coined this as part of the savior complex, describing a compulsive need to rescue others at the expense of one's own well-being. This pattern, linked to codependency, can create an unhealthy dynamic where your self-worth becomes tied to fixing others' problems.

Being kind and helping others is, of course, a good thing; however, not to the point where your need to take care of others is bigger than the need to take care of yourself. Back then, I thought I was just being a good person. I didn't realize that my need to help others was coming from my desperate desire to feel needed, valued, and good about myself.

No matter how many times I went out of my way to please and help others, I still didn't feel whole or complete. It felt like a never-ending cycle, and as I got older, the desire to feel good about myself seemed to grow with me. I never really paid attention to my feelings or needs, so it was easier for me to focus on what other people wanted. It gave me a sense of purpose and made me feel better about myself; it was as if I was confirming to the world that I was useful.

The truth is that when you realize your own worth and value, you don't feel the need to prove it to anyone because it's something you know at the very core of your being. Trying to prove to the world and to myself that I was useful felt like I was trying to fill up a bucket of water that had a hole at the bottom of it. It fills up for a few seconds, and before you know it, it's empty once again.

Having these kinds of personality traits puts you in a vulnerable position. If you're as naive as I was, you fail to realize that other people are not like you. You don't realize that other people might have bad intentions and try to take advantage of your neediness to help others. I learned this lesson the hard way. After years of neglecting and ignoring my own needs and prioritizing other people's happiness before mine, I found myself depleted of energy and completely out of touch with what I needed and who I was.

INSIGHTFUL LESSON: When the need to take care of others is bigger than the need to take care of yourself, it's not called kindness, it's called self-sabotage.

One of the scariest moments that hit me hard after I broke up with my narcissist happened when I was sitting in my bed, trying to figure out what to watch on YouTube or Netflix. For weeks, I opened up my laptop and stared blankly at the screen. I realized that I didn't even know what kind of movies or shows I enjoyed watching. This made me feel panicked. I remember asking myself: *"What's wrong with me? Why am I not able to type one single word in the search bar to look for something that I am interested in?"*

This is such a perfect and painful example of what happens to people after a narcissistic relationship. They feel completely hollow and wonder, "What is my truth? What is the Truth? Who am I?" Their eyes are glazed over, their stance is dissociated, as if they are drugged, but they are not drugged; their sense of self is annihilated. It's a psychic lobotomy of sorts, where they have no grounding in SELF. To compound this, they may no longer have a connection to their life before the narcissist, which leaves them more disconnected from who they really are.

The more I focused on the fear that I was feeling, the more paralyzed I got. So, I started asking myself how and why this was happening. Looking back at our relationship, he always used to choose what movie or show to watch together. He never asked me what I would like to watch, and when I rarely suggested something in the beginning of our relationship, he shut it down immediately or made fun of my suggestions.

You must understand that this starts as a normal response to either wanting to please a partner, being amenable and open, and a sense that time together (abandonment fears) is more valued than Netflix preferences. This erosion of the Self happens slowly, with intermittent seductions and control tactics. Grace's Netflix example encompasses a long identity disintegration wherein the narcissist capitalizes on the Empath's wounds and kind heart as a strategy. People on the "outside" who only see the end result, per se, don't understand the insidious nature of the degradation the victim or Empath endures, braided with moments of seduction and even tenderness.

I realized that the crisis I was going through was bigger than just not knowing what to watch on Netflix. It reflected how out of touch I was with myself and who I really was. For so many years, I had never asked myself what I wanted to do, where I wanted to go, what I liked doing, or who I wanted to be. I just followed him and let him decide everything for me. My lack of self-worth and the inability to identify my needs and express them forced me to see myself through him.

After a few weeks of despair, I built up the courage to type a few keywords in the search bar. The only way to find out what I liked was to try to discover what stimulated my brain. As simple as that sounds, it was not easy. I had to work through feelings of shame and embarrassment for what I liked to watch. I had to learn how to give myself permission and let myself know that it is okay to be curious about topics which he didn't follow.

Learning what interests me was more enjoyable than I ever thought, and it encouraged me to embark on a journey of self-discovery. For the first time ever, I started feeling like I was developing a sense of identity that belonged to me and no one else.

I call this the "me of me." Spiritually, I posit that it's our inner being/higher self/God that sends us these divine urges that feel enlivening, creative, and personal. The "divine urge" is what kept tugging at her to speak up, to fight, and to question; as she detoxified and detangled from him, the divine urge became more playful, original, and productive. I hold that the psychotherapeutic process—after cleaning up the traumatic wounds and learning coping tools to calm the central nervous system—is about mining for the divine urges that make the person uniquely themselves. I call this process the bridge from trauma surviving into trauma rising. Grace's book is an example of this very bridge, tools, and processes included.

And from then onwards, I started being more curious about other aspects of myself. Getting to know myself helped me break through my codependency as I was able to recognize my strengths, my interests, and which direction I wanted to take in life.

Not knowing who you are, what you like, and what you enjoy doing are symptoms of codependency. The first time I started reading about codependency, I couldn't deny how perfectly it described who I was. And apparently, there are many people out there struggling with similar issues. It's been estimated that 90% of the American population has codependent behavior. Research carried out by Crester and Lombardo (1999) found that nearly half of the nation's college students surveyed showed codependent personality traits.

It makes perfect sense that the college student has codependent traits, especially today in the era of social media. One way to understand codependency is with an image of a permeable wall between the inner and outer world. It is natural for humans to imitate other humans; it is, in fact, an adaptive, evolutionary trait that helps us learn systemic and societal norms in order to survive in the ecosystems into which we are born.

Neuroscientifically speaking, humans are born with "mirror neurons," which are very specific neurons located in the premotor cortex that serve to respond and/or imitate the actions we see in other humans. If we don't have a strong sense of self, which most of us don't at a college age, it is easy to mimic others, mimic our culture, and mimic the systems that surround us. We can thus see why constant messaging from social media can confuse and create a sense of self that is based on mimicry rather than a genuine exploration of the unique urge within each of us. Hence, my personal and professional emphasis and insistence on using modalities that lead us to the inner journey of self-discovery. When we are solidifying our internal nature via personal urge, we can interact with our external world with a stronger psychological perimeter (boundaries) without getting swept away by narcissists or by societal mimicry. Co-dependence is basically a permeable identity wall that has gone askew.

Common codependency traits include:

- Feeling responsible for other people's feelings and well-being
- Have strong people-pleasing tendencies
- Experience feelings of anxiety and guilt when others have a problem
- Feeling compelled to help others fix their problems
- Smothering others with affection, gifts, or gestures of goodwill
- Feeling bored and empty if they don't help others
- Having difficulty describing who they are, what they enjoy doing, and what they like
- Neglecting themselves and prioritizing others
- Difficulty expressing needs, emotions, and asserting boundaries
- Emotionally dependent on their partners
- Seeking validation and feelings of self-worth outside of themselves

A combination of these codependency traits makes up the perfect bait for a narcissist. Narcissists seek people who are ready to meet their needs at all costs. They recognize that they are extremely demanding and that not everyone is willing to meet their unrealistic expectations. On the other hand, codependents are always seeking to help and please others. Voila, you have the perfect match.

Narcissists are the takers and manipulators, and codependents are the givers and pleasers. The roles they play in the relationship seem natural to them because they have been practicing them their entire lives. Codependents naturally give up their power due to their submissive nature, and narcissists thrive on control and power, so their roles are perfectly coordinated.

Grace describes this relational dynamic beautifully! The narcissist literally "plugs into" the codependent like a socket. Per my teachings, the co-dependent is interchangeable with the wounded Empath, as most wounded Empaths are co-dependent because of their ability to feel environments and intrinsic impulse to harmonize them, which distorts into extreme people-pleasing or fawning. As Grace says, what a perfect match for the narcissistic usurper!

The relationship between narcissists and codependents is highly turbulent and full of drama. Despite their chaotic, turbulent relationship, these dysfunctional compatible partners find it difficult to break up, and their relationship can last for many years. Narcissists present themselves as having high self-esteem, and codependents fail to pick up on their need for external validation at the beginning of the relationship. So, narcissists need codependents to feed their ego and stabilize their self-esteem, while codependents need to feel needed and valued, so they sacrifice their own needs to please the narcissist.

The dance between narcissists and codependents can go on for years. Codependency and NPD are disorders of the self. Unless either one of them decides to work on their relationship with themself, it will be almost impossible to end the relationship. Even though it is challenging to overcome codependency and let go of the need to please others, a codependent has a higher chance of working on themself than a narcissist due to the nature of narcissistic personality disorder.

Indeed, NPD and codependency are disorders of the Self, and what gets lost inside the narcissistic mirage is that the narcissist has even less of a sense of self than the co-dependent. It looks like the co-dependent is the slave and the narcissist is the master, and yet, without the co-dependent to serve and supply the narcissist, the narcissist doesn't exist. Please excuse my language here as I use it for dramatic and strategic purposes.

This relational dynamic has existed historically in governments, politics, corporate bureaucracies, and economic structures. Without the co-dependent supply—i.e., those who feel lowly on the societal hierarchy, generally who have more need, and who will thus tolerate unequal dynamics—the narcissistic system collapses. The narcissist needs the co-dependent to stay wounded in order to exist.

Breaking free from codependency can help you realize that to be valued, loved, and appreciated, you don't need to sacrifice your own happiness and needs for others. Putting yourself first will feel unnatural in the beginning. But as you start working on the relationship with yourself, you'll realize how much you were missing out on. Knowing and engaging in activities that set your soul on fire is way more powerful and enjoyable than pleasing others for the sake of being valued and accepted.

The healing process from codependency is a challenging one, yet extremely liberating. Through self-love and self-reliance, you learn how to move away from toxic and narcissistic relationships and move towards interdependent and loving relationships.

Grace's description here of the dynamic, the journey, and the answer out of codependency is nothing less than sublime. Knowing and solidifying the self, via inner exploration, with psychic injuries and psychic preferences, automatically constructs a WHOLE self and repels boundary violators.

Self-Reflective Exercise

What are my emotional needs? (Ex: affection, connection, security, autonomy.)

How do I nourish my emotional needs? (Ex: spending time with family/friends, utilizing my skills, and building authentic relationships.)

What are my physical needs? (Ex: healthy food, good sleep, physical exercise, sexual stimulation.)

How do I nourish my physical needs? (Ex: preparing healthy meals, sleeping 8 hours a day, working out.)

What are my mental needs? (Ex: clarity, calm, cognitive stimulation.)

How do I nourish my mental needs? (Ex: spending time alone, taking a break, learning a new skill.)

What are my spiritual needs? (Ex: inner peace, fulfillment, joy.)

How do I nourish my spiritual needs? (Ex: meditation, journaling, music, art, yoga.)

Meditation, or the practice of going inside to listen and observe, is a powerful way of listening to wants and needs. In Dynamic, we use a specific meditation that I call the "Wanting Meditation." It is common for co-dependents and wounded Empaths to feel ashamed of their wants because they have been ridiculed for them, demeaned, or they have reached desperate levels of wanting.

In the "Wanting Meditation" (remembering the mechanical approach of energy releasing), we say yes to wanting, and even more so, desperate wanting. We locate where the wanting is lodged in our bodies, head, chest, stomach, and even genitals. We visualize the "wanting" energy accumulated there. We imagine a release valve like an open window, an open door, or an actual valve through which the energy will go through.

I encourage folks to use yeshales (saying "yesssss" with the exhale) while visualizing the energy leaving the body. Repeat the process over and over, until it feels less desperate, quieter, or lighter. What's essential here is not to shame or demean what you want—let's say a desperate need to be married or to have money—because it's signaling something about your true self. What this process does is calm the emotional torment and validate it. Once wants and needs are calibrated through acceptance, they will transmute into preferences, and preferences automatically become boundaries. Bam! Once you know and validate your preferences, you are protected because you can walk away, state them, and get them.

It may seem odd that the most precise way to establish boundaries is by knowing what you need, want, and prefer. In healthy family systems—or any system for that matter—needs, wants, and preferences are seen, heard, and most importantly, RESPECTED. In an atmosphere of respect, boundaries do not have to be fought for or insisted upon because respect paves the way for mutual agreement. Most co-dependents, trauma survivors, wounded Empaths, and addicts have absolutely no clue about their true wants, needs, or preferences because they were either serving the needs of the adult others, were actively obliterated (as in the case of narcissistic environments), or were completely neglected.

Wants and needs show up spastically in the forms of addictions and wounded relationships but not directly. Because these "apparitions" of wants and needs are in the midst of hurtful and demeaning conditions, they are infused with self-doubt and shame and struggle to reach the status of preferences and boundaries. The co-dependent will always be trumped by the narcissist because they are crystal clear on what they want and need. Having said that, even when not blurry, our higher Self or beautiful internal being does show up, notwithstanding, in the form of a guttural "NO" or "YES" to help us know that a line has been crossed. Yes, these lines get crossed and crossed and therefore become indistinguishable, but sometimes, we can hear the "NO" or "YES" of a preference.

Five Behavioral Changes to Stop Being Codependent with a Narcissist

#1. Stop focusing on how to help the narcissist. Accept the fact that no amount of unconditional love, empathy, or acceptance can heal them.

#2. Focus on yourself. How much time and energy did you spend thinking about how to help the narcissist? Shift that energy and focus on how to help yourself. Take some time in a quiet place and reflect on what you would like to do. If you don't know where to start, just give it a shot and see what happens. It's the only way to find out what you like or dislike.

- What makes you happy?
- How do you like to spend your time?
- What goals do you have in life?
- What would you like to achieve?
- Are there any hobbies or activities you have wanted to try?

#3. Stop seeking validation from others and learn to seek joy from within. Relying on others to feel valued, loved, and good about yourself puts you in a very vulnerable position. By learning who you are and what gives you joy, you take the power back over how you feel. This helps you feel empowered and self-reliant.

#4. Identify your needs and learn how to nourish them. In the previous self-reflective exercise, you had to fill in your emotional, physical, mental, and spiritual needs. As a codependent, you are an expert at nurturing others. Direct your nurturing tendencies towards yourself. To achieve holistic balance and to feel whole, you must learn how to take care of yourself first.

#5. Practice self-love and self-care. When was the last time you did something nice for yourself? And when was the last time you did something nice for others? Codependents have so much love to give to others, but they don't know how to provide some of that love to themselves. Self-love is key to breaking free from codependency.

Write down these 'Free From Codependency' affirmations and put the paper somewhere you can see it every day. Ex: on the bathroom mirror so you can read them every day while brushing your teeth. Repeating affirmations helps you reprogram your subconscious mind through your conscious mind:

- "I love you, [Your Name]."
- "I am worthy of love and acceptance."
- "I take care of my needs."
- "My needs and feelings matter."
- "I take care of others, but I take care of myself first."

Chapter 10

Low Self-Esteem & Self-Worth

WHEN I STARTED SEEING my ex, I didn't perceive myself as someone with low self-esteem. I felt good about myself and was confident in social settings. If someone had told me I had low self-esteem, I would have laughed in disbelief. However, when it came to self-worth, that was a different story.

Although self-esteem and self-worth are often used interchangeably, they play distinct roles in shaping our identity and self-perception. Nowadays, there is a growing awareness of these concepts. Many people can define them, discuss them, and even advocate for their importance. Yet, despite this increasing awareness, countless individuals continue to struggle with truly embodying their self-worth or maintaining a healthy level of self-esteem.

The truth is, there is a profound difference between intellectually understanding these concepts and deeply integrating them into our lives. Our actions, choices, and behaviors ultimately reveal what we truly believe about ourselves. So, what's the difference between these two terms?

Self-esteem is more externally influenced—it's how you perceive yourself in relation to your actions, abilities, and social interactions. It is shaped by your achievements, social skills, confidence levels, and the way others respond to you. A person with high self-esteem generally believes in their capabilities and feels competent in various areas of life. However, self-esteem can fluctuate based on external validation, success, or failure. It is tied to what you do and how well you do it.

Self-worth, on the other hand, is internal and intrinsic—it is the fundamental belief that you are valuable simply because you exist. Self-worth is not determined by achievements, external validation, or social status. It is about recognizing and embracing yourself in your entirety—flaws, imperfections, and all. Self-worth is the unwavering truth that you are worthy of love, respect, and dignity, just as any other living being is. It is the foundation upon which everything else is built.

Grace makes such an important distinction here that may still seem hazy for anyone still healing or swirling from narcissistic abuse. Behavioral examples can be more helpful in distinguishing the two, and Grace proceeds to show just that. Tracking concrete examples in your journal also helps with real and tangible examples that aid in disentangling from the narcissistic haze or mirage, where self-doubt reigns.

Both self-esteem and self-worth are essential pillars of mental health and self-perception. Suppose you have solid self-worth but low self-esteem. In that case, you may feel inherently valuable as a human being, yet still struggle with self-doubt, imposter syndrome, or constant comparison to others, ultimately holding yourself back from reaching your full potential. On the other hand, if you lack self-worth, you may find yourself drawn to individuals who reinforce the deep-seated belief that you are unworthy and not good enough.

Looking back at my relationships, it seems like the universe was on a mission to teach me a lesson so I could learn what it means to know your self-worth. The narcissist picked up on that, too. He could sense that my self-esteem was solid. So, every time he verbally abused me, he specifically and strategically targeted my weak point: my self-worth. Narcissists know exactly how to push your buttons, so they will attack you on your weaknesses and insecurities to disempower you. They eat you from the inside, stripping your confidence away bit by bit to feed on your pain.

At the beginning of the relationship, he was always complimenting me and telling me all sorts of things a girl likes to hear. He presented himself as above standard, confident, intelligent, and highly charismatic. I felt humbled and honored that someone like him was interested in me. And that was the first indication that I had no idea of how worthy I was as a human being. My actions and behaviors showed him very clearly that I put him on a pedestal, which is exactly how he wanted to be treated.

Anything that feels like a pedestal, whether towards you or towards them, is worth looking at, especially early on, as it may be a red flag. The symbolism of a pedestal intrinsically describes a hierarchical difference, a distance based on superior/inferior dynamics. Some good self-reflection questions are "Do I feel that they are superior to me or better than me? Do I feel superior or better than them? Why?" and list the answers. Even if not in a narcissistic relationship, poking at this sensation early on is a worthy endeavor as it may provide answers to address your own self-worth.

I made him feel good about himself, feeding him with narcissistic supply as I was bending backwards to attend to his needs and make him happy in every way possible. Anyone who feels whole and knows their self-worth wouldn't drop whatever they were doing to rush to their partner the moment they ask to meet. This kind of behavior gives out the wrong message. In my case, my ex quickly realized that my world revolved around him, and he immediately took advantage of that.

"Dropping everything" is another good example that may signal abandonment fears, fawning, and anxiety, rather than eager excitement for a new love. A good question here is "what does it feel like to not respond as soon as possible? Does it bring up abandonment issues or fear that they'll be upset? What does it feel like to ask them to wait? Is it anxiety-provoking, does it feel like "you'll get in trouble," does it feel scary to not please?" The answers can indicate co-dependence, PTSD, and underneath all of the above, low self-worth.

It makes perfect sense for narcissists to target people with low self-esteem and low self-worth. People with low self-esteem tend to question their own behavior before they question the behavior of others. Unfortunately, they end up taking responsibility for other people's mistakes, which is the perfect situation for a narcissist. Individuals with low self-worth are more likely to struggle with self-reliance, and narcissists intentionally make their partners dependent on them. So, they get tricked into believing that the narcissist can provide them with experiences or could help them achieve things they couldn't imagine achieving by themselves.

Grace makes several points here that signal childhood issues. First, although it is important to be able to keep an open mind about our beliefs or competencies to stay in a learning demeanor, when we immediately succumb to the influence of others, it is a way we subjugate ourselves to someone else's interpretation of things. It is likely that as a child, opinions, insights, or learnings were dismissed, disregarded, and possibly not even acknowledged. Parental responses such as, "I can see you were thoughtful about that," "I can see your point of view," or, for smaller children,

"Good thinking!" "Let's try it your way then we can try it mine," are all validating experiences of an emerging Self. The underlying message is "What you think matters," and the parent is not the only one who can think in the room.

The habit of self-doubting or self-questioning and relegating all authority to another is just that, a long-term psychological pattern. Second, it is very common in a conflict-ridden home, a home with a controlling parent, or a tension-filled, silent home, for the child to blame themselves for what is occurring. This is a survival response. The child cannot blame or be angry at the adult caregivers, not only because there is an inherent expectation that the adult knows better, but also because the adults are the ones who provide us with survival scaffoldings such as shelter, food, and physical or emotional care.

Psychoanalytically speaking, the child's psyche perceives going against the human who provides them with survival safety and a sense of self as a death. This is a non-verbal, deeply unconscious belief that can multiply into other attachment relationships if left unhealed. The path to healing is recognizing it once it has been triggered in a relationship, as Grace is doing here. It's much easier to manipulate someone who puts them on a pedestal and is ready to give up everything to make them happy. Narcissists can identify these traits and characteristics in our personalities, as they are like predators hunting for vulnerable people. Having low self-esteem or low self-worth is definitely a vulnerability that narcissists use to their advantage.

If you have a history of abuse, trauma, bullying, or identity issues, you're more likely to develop self-esteem and self-worth issues. This means that you need to be more careful and that it is essential to work on these traumas prior to getting into further relationships. If you try to rush into another relationship, it's highly likely that you will meet another narcissist and repeat the same cycle all over again.

The mind likes patterns and learns to identify them quickly; these neurological patterns can be called neural pathways, psychological schemas, attachment styles, neuroassociations, among others. It is also an unconscious survival program to gravitate to what is familiar. What is familiar can sometimes be a mirage for safety, but in actuality, it is not if you come from an abusive, addictive, neglectful, or dysfunctional home. The adult child of an alcoholic may feel immediately attracted to the only alcoholic at a party; this doesn't often occur on a conscious level, but is rather like a heat-seeking missile that is activated when these neuroassociations—comprised of memory, sensations, and emotions—light up when they recognize what is familiar.

When Grace described having very strong feelings for him when she first met him, on a conscious level, these feelings include a natural attraction to anyone who is charismatic, but they also include that huge unconscious iceberg below the surface that reminded her of an attachment figure or several. Knowing your attachment style and why you have them is an extremely helpful tool for your healing, but also for picking your next partner. This moves the unconscious decision-making into the conscious and allows choice discernment, even when you feel instinctively very attracted to someone.

Narcissists and people with low self-worth have something in common. They subconsciously try to feel better by finding partners that reflect the perfect mirror image of themselves. The narcissist wants special treatment, and a person with low self-esteem and self-worth wants to feel valued and needed. Narcissists want servants, and people with low self-esteem or lack of self-worth are more likely to develop a need to please and serve others.

What Grace describes here is that plug and socket type of attraction; the narcissist and the person with low self-worth—or the wounded Empath—are a perfect fit. However, the mirage that the Narcissist constructs with great strategy and precision is that the wounded individual cannot live without the narcissist and needs him/her to survive, when all along, it is the narcissist who feels completely non-existent without the supply of these wounded "servers." It is why narcissists often are unfaithful or seem like "players" because they juggle multiple relationships, keeping the flame alive in all of them, in order to maintain an endless stream of supply that they clearly cannot give themselves because they feel utterly empty if left alone.

At the beginning of the relationship, both narcissists and people with low self-esteem try to impress each other by inflating their skills or qualities. They're both intending to present their best ideal self to each other. Intending to inflate one's skills or qualities shows that you subconsciously fear and believe that you will be rejected if you show your authentic self.

As you get closer to a narcissist, you realize that they were just wearing a mask to hide their deep-seated lack of self-worth. The problem arises when their partner starts seeing their vulnerable parts, fearing that they will be rejected, and that they will be seen as imposters pretending to be someone they're not. Just to make it clear, no level of acceptance and unconditional love can resolve this. It's a cycle that keeps repeating itself because they truly feel endangered in their own self-worth.

Indeed, this statement is not an exaggeration; the narcissist will not do the work of going inside themselves because of their terror of finding nothing or of discovering the self-hate they carry. The narcissist's defense is textbook classic as they project onto others their own experience of nothingness and self-hate. These projections are extremely powerful and cause severe damage, as we see in Grace's example. Can you see why children, people with kind hearts, and people with low self-esteem/worth are perfect targets? The narcissist needs a receptacle to put their rage and chronic existential emptiness into.

As a result, they refuse to be real, become distant to avoid being intimate and open themselves up to you, and try to maintain the relationship at a superficial level. A narcissist can stay in a relationship as long as their partner makes them feel that they're perfect and flawless, because this makes them feel safe. When the relationship starts getting deeper, they panic because they can't bear the downgraded value of themselves when it starts to be reflected in the relationship.

It is true that the narcissist increases their destructive tactics once "discovered" by publicly smearing the person, privately demeaning them, emotionally, and physically abusing them. They may also find other sources of supply (as he did when they were on vacation) to both regenerate themselves and to inflict damage.

It is worth noting that what is most common is that the narcissist is never the "abandoner" in the long-term, even when they constantly threaten to abandon; it is very difficult to rid oneself of the narcissist, which is why the "no contact" policy is strongly recommended after breaking free from them. No contact is extremely painful and an arduous process that requires intense recovery and a commitment to healing above anything else, especially when it comes to a narcissist parent or family member. Be thus forewarned, it is generally not the narcissist who leaves or ends things. This feels like one is loved if one has a fear of abandonment. This is not love; this is narcissistic supply. It is the wounded person or Empath who must heal and end things. Full stop.

Narcissists want to think of themselves as omnipotent beings, and their ego can't bear the self-image that is being reflected back to them in a relationship. They want to continue seeing the admiration and respect in the eyes of their partners, and they cannot bear someone looking at them with compassion, empathy, or interest in a wounded past. The more their partners try to nurture their emotional injuries, the more repulsed they feel and continue to pull back to avoid the emotional turbulence and discomfort triggered within themselves.

Foolishly so, that's exactly what I tried to do when I realized that he had his own emotional wounds, which were clearly unresolved. I used to feel compassion for him, and I felt the need to help him. I thought that by showing him unconditional love and acceptance, regardless of his flaws and vulnerabilities, I would help him heal. However, he refused to accept any of it. Accepting my attempts to nourish his wounds would have made him focus on his wounds and thus acknowledge that he is not perfect or omnipotent. To feel superior again, he used to attack my insecurities by using belittling and degrading comments. The weaker my self-esteem got and the lower my self-worth fell, the more power he got over me.

Let's underscore a few things here about caring for wounds. For any caring human, it is logical to feel compassion and to want to help someone who comes from a wounded past or who has a wound; it is a natural human response to care. I posit that the intrinsic human characteristic of caring for other humans is what has kept our species alive. Whether it be through physical wounds or emotional ones, humans caring for other humans have developed healing modalities, missions that have saved entire ethnic and racial groups, liberation movements, and provided sanctuaries for those in the greatest need. Caring is a natural human trait that the narcissist has amputated, which leads me to the second point about wounds and caring vis-à-vis the narcissist.

The etiology of narcissistic personality disorder begins with a wound (or several)—actually entitled "the narcissistic wound"—that was so egregious the narcissist had to amputate their caring function entirely in order to survive. Caring likely caused an inordinate amount of pain and terror in them as children but also did not provide any relief from the harm with which they were inflicted, and conceivably made it worse. Even as one reads this, a natural instinct to feel compassion for the narcissist is a worthy human response. Caring for and helping someone who is wounded is evolutionarily adaptive. Where this instinct goes completely awry with the narcissist is that the narcissist refuses—not chooses—but refuses to look inside themselves to heal and therefore is in a repetitive cycle of destruction that pulls anyone who wants to help them. The narcissist and the wounded person or Empath may begin their lives with a similar story of profound wounding, but their paths will drastically diverge when the wounded Empath—like Grace—will courageously look inside and begin the healing process to liberate themselves.

A common tactic by narcissists to attack our self-esteem is withholding intimacy from their partners. It took me a while to realize what was happening. I was in so much pain that I couldn't think clearly and notice the well-strategized manipulative technique. He used to spend all day giving me all kinds of sweet talk and telling me how he couldn't wait to get back home and make love to me. However, when he came home, he used to start teasing me with his words and then just shrug off his shoulders and reject me. Out of nowhere, he used to tell me that he was not feeling it and locked himself away in his bedroom for a couple of nights.

Every time he shrugged his shoulders and rejected me, he made me feel like there was something wrong with me. This happened countless times, and I felt sick to my stomach the moment I realized what he was doing. It took me months to become aware of this pattern and his malicious motive behind it. He intentionally tried to make me feel unwanted and rejected to continue breaking what was left of my self-esteem. I started reading and learning about this kind of emotional abuse, and I learned that narcissists withhold intimacy from their partners either to punish them or to keep them hooked on them, craving their love and affection.

This withholding of intimacy is the exact opposite of care; it is cruelty.

The more I learned about what was happening, the more I realized how pathological he was. I started accepting the fact that it was impossible to have a healthy, loving relationship with someone who was narcissistic. So, I started reading about what a healthy relationship looks like, and it sounded the complete opposite of the kind of relationship that I was in.

To develop a fulfilling relationship, it always requires being authentic and taking off masks. A relationship isn't about being superior to one another; it's about moving forward and growing together from a place of truth. Showing your authentic self with all your flaws and imperfections makes you feel vulnerable, and it is essential to build true intimacy with a partner who makes you feel safe. If you already struggle with self-esteem and self-worth, getting involved with a narcissist will leave you feeling less worthy than ever before. The only way to break free from this kind of toxic relationship is to work on the relationship with yourself. Once you build up your confidence and realize your self-worth, you'll become self-reliant and realize that you can achieve anything you want on your own.

In a way, we can choose to see these experiences as mirrors, reflecting what needs healing within us. Rather than mere suffering, they can be viewed as an unpleasant, distasteful medicine, bringing buried wounds to the surface and allowing us to transform them into strength. By reframing these challenges, we shift from a victim mindset to one of empowerment, bringing forth the magician archetype. We become able to see beyond pain and use it as fuel for growth and transformation. In doing so, we become alchemists of our own lives, transforming our struggles into wisdom, resilience, and a deeper sense of self-worth.

INSIGHTFUL LESSON: Believing that the narcissist is giving you something you can't have on your own is an illusion. What you seek in others already exists within you. You are more resourceful than you think. As the poet Rumi wisely said, "You are not a drop in the ocean, but the ocean in a drop."

How to Boost Your Self-Confidence?

#1. Make a list of your achievements. Focus on your achievements. Don't get stuck on what didn't work, and celebrate small victories.

___

___

___

___

#2. Count your blessings. Acknowledge and embrace your blessings. When we're stressed, it's common to take things for granted. Remind yourself of the positive things, no matter how small or irrelevant they might seem.

#3. Shift self-negative talk to self-empowerment talk. How we speak to ourselves is a major factor that will help you boost your confidence. Sometimes, we don't even realize how we speak to ourselves, especially after listening to belittling and degrading comments about ourselves. Replace each negative thought with a positive affirmation. Repeat, repeat, repeat!

#4. Challenge yourself, learn something new. When we learn something new, we feel empowered and boost our self-esteem. Challenging ourselves also helps us to build self-confidence as we remind ourselves of our strengths and capabilities.

#5. Take care of yourself. It's important that you take good care of yourself so you feel good about yourself. This means eating nourishing food, doing physical exercise, getting enough sleep, and taking care of your self-image. It's difficult to feel confident if you don't feel comfortable in your own skin.

#6. Learn how to accept compliments. If you have low self-esteem, it's highly likely that you don't know how to accept positive feedback and compliments. Perhaps you think people are making fun of you when they praise you. Or maybe you shrink yourself and play small, believing that accepting compliments or owning your strengths makes you arrogant. But true humility isn't about rejecting your qualities. It's about acknowledging them without ego. Learn to accept compliments and embrace them, and start complimenting yourself more!

#7. Surround yourself with good people. Having people who love you, support you, and uplift you will bring out the best in you. Surround yourself with people who help you grow and become a better person.

The Differences Between Self-Esteem & Self-Worth

SELF-ESTEEM	SELF-WORTH
Actions What actions are you taking? Ex: *apply for a promotion*	**Identity** Who are you? Ex: *a spiritual being having a human experience*
Self-Representation How do you present yourself? Ex: *confident & outspoken*	**Morality** Are your life choices aligned with your morals and values? Ex: *my life choices align with love, respect, kindness*
External Self-Image How do you think that others perceive you? Ex: *kind, courageous*	**Truth** Do you express your thoughts, needs & opinions? Ex: *sharing my opinion, expressing my needs*
Comparison Do you compare yourself to others? Ex: *comparing myself to people who are better/worse than me*	**Living as You** Do you live authentically? Ex: *are you authentic in how you present yourself & communicate with others?*

What actions will I take in the next three months to build up my self-esteem and self-confidence?

ACTION	INITIAL DATE	FREQUENCY	WHY?	WHAT & HOW?
What action do I need to take?	When will I start?	How many times a week?	For which purpose am I doing this?	What will I learn & how will this benefit me?

Chapter 11

Inner Core Beliefs

I USED TO THINK THAT I was just unlucky when it came to relationships. I didn't realize that I was also accountable for my disastrous romantic stories. My actions and choices were dictated by my subconscious beliefs, and these beliefs manifested themselves in my relationships.

Accepting the fact that I chose to stay in an abusive relationship wasn't easy. After all, it wasn't my fault that someone took advantage of my kindness and compassion. Nevertheless, things for me really started to change when I realized that even though I was doing it unconsciously, I was manifesting my reality.

There are several ways to talk about manifestation, which is commonly understood as our intrinsic ability to not only create our life reality, but also that our life until now was created by us and stems from our conscious, and mostly, unconscious beliefs. These beliefs were deposited into us as children by our caregivers, community, religion, ethnicity, race, etc. It follows then that our adult relational approaches are a myriad of learned beliefs that we play out on "automatic." We can see why manifestation is a controversial belief in itself in that, given some horrific childhood experiences or traumatic life events, one would question how one created those realities.

From a very watered-down neuroscientific perspective, as children we form neural pathways or neuroassociations—a complex web of neural connections that are strung together by cognitions, emotions, and sensations—that are reinforced by experiences. Commonly stated in the neuroscientist community, "The more we fire, the more we wire," meaning that these neural pathways become more rigidly bound over time if re-experienced. Ironically and simultaneously, these neural pathways (beliefs) form a filter of sorts, or a perspective, based on these specific experiences and hence perpetuate a reenactment of those beliefs, which in turn, create what an individual experiences as their reality.

INSIGHTFUL LESSON: Whether you're conscious of it or not, you're manifesting your life through your inner world map and everyday choices. By no means am I saying that I deserved the abuse or that it's justifiable. But owning my responsibility helped me reclaim my power in my life as I realized that I was in the driver's seat. Instead of perceiving myself as a helpless victim, I perceived myself as an active participant who had a choice in this story.

Whether one believes that one is responsible for what is manifesting in one's life or not, what Grace describes here—seeing herself as an active participant in her life story—is paramount. Once she acknowledges that she pilots her life and has agency over it, in spite of her wounds, past trauma, or derailed decisions, Grace becomes the creator of her story.

In Cognitive Behavioral Therapy, these are called schemas. It is a deep-rooted cognitive framework from which we organize and understand our reality. Schemas are a way we make sense of our environment, even in painful and disorganized situations; they can provide a semblance of relief and normalcy because they help us interpret a life experience. These schemas form into defenses, patterns, and sometimes distortions that become a way of navigating the world. An example of a distorted schema is when a child is in a conflict-ridden home with an unhappy caregiver; the child can develop the schema that it is their fault that their caregiver is unhappy and that they are to blame for the family conflict. The defenses this can engender are for the child to be "extra good," or be "the fixer or savior" in the home. As an adult, this can translate into being attracted to conflict situations or individuals and replay the role of savior or fixer. This scenario is extremely common for wounded Empaths, particularly because their significant and default characteristic is to harmonize environments. The more deeply rooted schema here is the unconscious wish that by playing this role or by being extra good, they will be loved.

How do these schemas or neural pathways become manifestations? Manifestations occur through what Gestalt psychology describes as the perceptual field. The perceptual field is the lens through which an individual sees life at a particular time. Even though there are multiple perceptual fields concurrently happening, we tend to go with the perceptual field that is most familiar and the one that has been repeated the most, i.e., hard-wired into our psyche. The lens through which we perceive life events stems from our past experiences and becomes a self-fulfilling prophecy, primarily because we will exclude other possibilities even if they co-exist.

Throughout my coaching sessions with my healer, I had several breakthroughs. I started questioning my beliefs to understand why I felt so scared to let go of such a toxic relationship and why I chose this guy in the first place. At that time, my self-esteem was completely broken, and I struggled to mention any positive skills or qualities that I had. I was paralyzed with fear as each and every time I looked within myself to mention something positive, I couldn't verbalize one single word.

The good news of doing our healing work is that over time, we begin to deconstruct our "given" schemas, perceptual fields, and beliefs, and we start to design new ones that are created and chosen by our healed SELF.

It thus follows that our perceptual field changes; when we scan the environment, we locate people, places, and things that fit our new identity, per se. In addition, our new schemas and beliefs—new mental models and/or neural pathways—manifest a new reality precisely because our "scanner" is not only seeking but visualizing an evolved version of what they were—voilà, manifestations in our external world! Quantum physics posits—and I butcher it a bit because I am not a quantum physicist—that the quantum field around us and between us holds constant waves of possibilities and depending upon where we set our gaze, per se, we collapse these waves into a material reality, i.e., what can be called a manifestation.

This parallels the gestalt notion that we co-exist within several realities, and we are the observers and the choosers of the reality that we are gazing upon. There are so many ways to discuss this, and they all converge on the premise that we can become the sovereign choosers and creators of the reality we live in, no matter what past we come from.

During our relationship, the narcissist used to start discussions where I felt like I was sitting for a job interview. He used to make me list down my skills and capabilities to prove to him that I was useful and to prove to him that I was worthy of his respect. At the time, I was so focused on finding answers to impress him that I didn't even realize how inappropriate these conversations were. He used to laugh at every skill that I mentioned, and shame me for not having any real useful skills or qualities. Initially, I didn't believe what he was saying, but after having the same conversation and arguments several times, I started to doubt myself. There was a point in my life when I felt like I wasn't able to do anything without him. I looked into my future and felt terrified at the thought of being without him; it felt like my life would end. I was completely under his spell, fooled by the insidious beliefs he had implanted in my head.

INSIGHTFUL LESSON: When you start seeing yourself as an active participant in your relationship, you reclaim your power back. You have a choice. Be brave. Take over the driver seat.

Breaking through my mental barriers wasn't easy. I started by challenging my beliefs to prove to myself that I was capable of learning and growing. I knew I had to face my demons to overcome the mess I had found myself in. So I started facing my fears, and I pushed myself to do the things that scared me the most. Each time I pushed through and overcame a challenge, I felt empowered and started letting go of what he made me believe about myself. I wanted to feel self-reliant, and I was willing to do everything in my power to break free from the suffering that I was going through.

Step by step, one challenge after the other, I managed to build up my confidence, and I started making different choices in life. I felt empowered, and I found the courage to continue moving forward with my transformation. Proving to myself that I had skills and capabilities wasn't enough to save me from my relationship. I knew that I had to go deeper and discover what I believed about myself that allowed me to tolerate abusive behavior from my partner. As I progressed in my healing journey, I realized that if I had known my self-worth and my value from the very beginning, I would have stopped the relationship much earlier.

This is such a beautiful description of Grace's commitment to deconstruct the inborn or hereditary schemas that were manifesting a reality she did not want. Her ability to self-observe and self-reflect, to stop herself from continuing down this destructive path, is a testament to the importance of the inner journey and the impact it has on the outer journey. Basically, as she tinkered with her internal patterns of low self-worth, she began to shift what was occurring to her externally, and of course, she felt empowered! We want results for the work we do, and this was giving her results, and results feel empowering.

Thanks to several moments of realization, I realized that I was holding on to him because I didn't believe in myself. My limiting beliefs about myself kept me stuck in the relationship. I bought into my own illusions derived from fear. I believed that by being with him, I could have the kind of life that I deeply desired. I failed to realize that he could never offer me what I needed and what I valued in a relationship. I saw myself through him, and even though the relationship was falling apart, I held on to the belief that it was better with him than without him. That's how strong our inner core beliefs are. Even when something is so obviously wrong for us, we go against what's right for us, driven by limiting beliefs that shape our reality.

A gentler way of approaching these limiting beliefs that create our reality is by realizing that they were first inherited, and then they became an unconscious habit. The process of making the unconscious conscious—what Grace is providing in this book—comes from observing our life and deciding whether it's what we want. Habit changing is challenging, but with guidance, support, coaching, and commitment, it's entirely possible and probable. Thank you, neuroplasticity, for giving us that hope and the high-level purpose for which to strive.

Our inner core beliefs act as our map of the world. They determine how we perceive ourselves and the world we live in. We filter and interpret our experiences through these core beliefs, which influence our decisions, relationships, behaviors, and how we interact with others.

For example, if a person has low self-esteem and someone gives them a genuine compliment, they might interpret the situation as someone trying to make fun of them. On the other hand, if a person is confident and someone gives them a compliment, they interpret the situation as someone complimenting them. So whatever beliefs you hold about yourself and the world around you affects how you interpret situations.

If you're not aware of these limiting beliefs, you mistake them to be the absolute truth. You end up making decisions based on the framework that you have in your mind. In reality they are your most deeply held assumptions based on previous experiences and influences. Inner core beliefs include automatic negative thoughts and they usually sound something like this:

- I am not good at...
- I can't do this because...
- Everyone thinks I'm...
- Nobody thinks I'm...
- I am not able to...
- I'll never be able to...
- I should fix the relationship because...

Try to catch yourself when you engage in this kind of self-negative talk and challenge those beliefs by questioning them. Check in with yourself to track down where the limiting belief comes from and what experience led you to buy into that belief. Most of our inner core beliefs are based on childhood assessments of our experiences which end up shaping who we become as adults. Throughout our life, we subconsciously attract evidence that affirms our inner core beliefs, and we repel anything that might challenge them. This is self-perpetuating and we end up creating our own reality and attracting people into our lives who continue to strengthen and reaffirm our beliefs. So, if at the very core of your being, you feel that you are not worthy or good enough, you will attract people like narcissists into your life who will continue to put you down and reflect what you think about yourself.

The good news is that core beliefs can be changed as we shed light on them and challenge these beliefs. Our ego doesn't like to be wrong, so we initially resist changing our beliefs or letting go of them. We expect external circumstances to change our beliefs and we fail to realize that we are victims of our own projections into our reality. But in order to start seeing different results, we need to start making different choices. And to start making different choices, we need to start thinking differently, and feeling differently.

When your internal world changes, it brings about change in your external world. Even though we like to think that we can control things in our external world, in reality the only power we have is over ourselves. Refusing to recognize and accept this will only cause more suffering as we keep trying to control outcomes or how other people feel about us. Why not change how we feel about ourselves?

Exactly! Why not change how we feel about ourselves? I repeat: the inner, healing, psychological, and spiritual journey is about getting a PhD on you, a most honorable endeavor.

INSIGHTFUL LESSON: As above, so below. As within, so without. This is the law of correspondence—your external reality is a direct reflection of your internal world.

How to Identify Limiting Beliefs

Step 1: Identify and write down some common thoughts, beliefs, and generalizations that you tell yourself. (Ex: I don't have what it takes… I don't have time… I don't deserve… I'm not good at…)

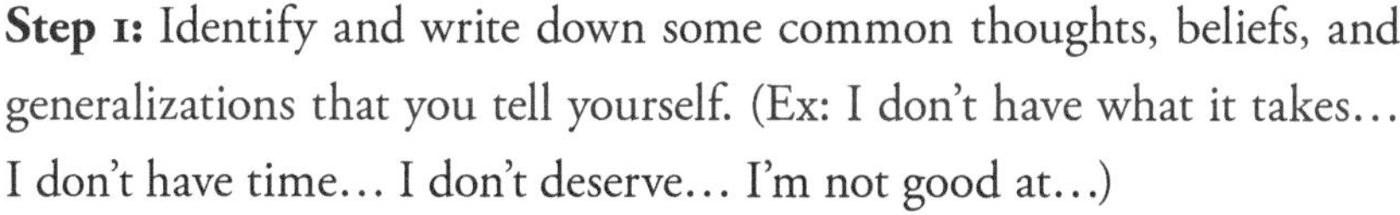

Step 2: Check in with yourself and see whether these statements about yourself are in your own voice or someone else's.

- When did you start believing this statement?
- Who influenced you to think like this?
- What experience influenced your thinking?

Step 3: Question and challenge your own way of thinking as much as you can.

Example: I don't have what it takes…

- Why don't you have what it takes?
- What have you tried so far?
- For how long did you try before you quit?
- What's really stopping you from going for it?

Example: I don't have time…

- How are you managing your time?
- What are your priorities?
- How can you manage your time better?
- How can you adjust your schedule to find time?

Example: I don't deserve…

- Says who?
- How do you know that you don't deserve it?
- Why don't you deserve it?
- What do I believe about myself that makes me feel this way?

There are so many processes and tools to identify limiting beliefs. Cognitive Behavioral Therapy (CBT), for example, is a highly effective, precise, and efficacious psychotherapeutic modality for identifying limiting beliefs and transforming them into more beneficial options.

My own Dynamic Meditation Method is based on being a portable and practical toolkit that can be done on the go and in real time. Beyond becoming daily meditators, Dynamic meditators are on-the-spot meditators. Sometimes our beliefs are chronically running in the background and we don't even know they are there, unconsciously steering our lives in all sorts of directions that we don't want. Let me offer two quick processes that will "pop" the unconscious or "pop" the limiting belief.

The first is to actually set a specific goal, for example, I'd like to lose 40 pounds in three months, or I'd like to make ten thousand dollars by a certain date. You will notice immediately the beliefs or obstacles that POP. Write them down! A very debilitating one can be But how?" Yes, it's a practical question, but it spirals most humans down a rabbit hole of despair and apathy. For now, set the goal and pop the unconscious, list the limiting beliefs, and observe them. You can then follow the steps in Grace's exercise to move into action.

The second suggestion is a holistic sequence of questions (Dynamic is based on self-inquiry meditations). Ask yourself: 'What do I want?' 'Now, what does my mind say about this?' (you can touch your forehead) 'What does my heart say?' (touch heart). 'What would my parents say?' etc.

Again, this is not to lock you into belief or to send you down a rabbit hole; it is a mechanical exercise to see what thoughts crowd your mind on a daily basis and likely drive you in misaligned directions. These two quick processes are just to pop the sequence. We do follow up with thought and feeling replacement sequences afterwards, but start here.

Generalizations, Self-Limitations & Assumptions

Generalizations and assumptions about the world you live in can take shape in the form of denial or describing how things are.

These usually sound like:

- '*True* love isn't real.'
- 'Love hurts.'
- 'It's impossible to meet someone better.'

I call these types of statements our internal formulas. Some examples are love=loss, happy=sad, more=less. These formulas are very dominant and have no doubt that they are controlling your approach to life. For example, love=loss is a formula we apply to falling in love. "When I fall in love, I'm always afraid of losing that person," or, "I'll lose them eventually." Happy=sad is when we get something we've always wanted or have a windfall of some sort, and believe that it will go wrong or wait for the "other shoe to drop."

Obviously, these beliefs are based on childhood experiences where these formulas were formed because of actual situations that did occur. In an alcoholic family or with a bipolar parent, when the alcoholic or parent was happy, the sense of trepidation was always high because soon enough, the mood would change, and maybe change drastically. Another formula here may be happy=scary. More=less is a formula I use to describe the feeling that when life is getting better it only means that there is a high price to pay for it or a sacrifice to make. I like replacing these formulas with new ones like more=more, happy=peaceful, love=more love. Again, these are simple visuals that make a strong impact on the mind. Breathing the new formulas into the body—what I call "depositing breaths"—is essential for re-memorizing new beliefs.

Self-limitations and assumptions are limiting beliefs imposed on ourselves or on other people that hold us back from growing and living a fulfilling life.

These can sound like:

- 'Others will laugh at me.'
- 'No one will believe me.'
- 'Everyone thinks I'm a failure.'
- 'Relationships should be like ....'

When you start digging into these beliefs to track them to their roots, you will realize that there is no truth behind them or that they aren't 100% entirely true. This realization will help you open your mind to new possibilities, new perspectives, and new choices that you couldn't access before. And that's when change starts to happen.

Changing our core beliefs is challenging and uncomfortable. You will need to learn how to be more comfortable with uncertainty as you challenge your usual way of thinking and step out of your comfort zone. It might be scary, as we naturally crave certainty and security as human beings. But it's much scarier knowing that your life will look like hell forever.

Chapter 12

Attachment Styles

MY DEAR SISTER WAS the first person that introduced me to the theory of attachment styles. For years, I used to argue with her, and I denied everything she was observing in my relationship dynamics. Even though it was extremely obvious, I just couldn't see it for myself. At the end of my relationship with my ex-narcissist, I surrendered. After 10 years of toxic and abusive relationships, I had to go deeper to understand how to break this pattern. If you have a pattern of attracting the same kind of toxic partners, your attachment style is probably one of the main reasons behind it.

Attachment theory was developed by John Bowlby and psychologist Mary Ainsworth back in the 1930s. According to the article on APA PsycNET (n.d.), our attachment style defines what kind of people we are attracted to and affects how we communicate and behave in relationships (The origins of attachment theory: John Bowlby and Mary Ainsworth. Developmental Psychology, 28(5), 759–775.). Identifying our attachment style can help us understand why we keep choosing similar partners and why we keep repeating the same patterns.

Attachment styles are comprehensive relational mental models, complex neural pathways, schemas, and/or inherited unconscious patterns. Attachment styles can be understood, healed, and calibrated with intention and care.

Just like most of our traumas, limiting beliefs, and insecurities, our attachment style is formed in our childhood. It all boils down to the emotional bond we form with our parents and caregivers when we were babies and young kids. Our early social experiences stimulate the development of the brain and act as a model for how to get our needs met. So if, as a kid, your parents or caregivers didn't know how to make you feel safe, secure, and protected, you might struggle with this later on in your romantic relationships. Suppose one or both parents were emotionally distant and you felt like you had to fight or strive for their love and affection. In that case, it will also affect how you behave in romantic relationships and what kind of partners you are attracted to at a subconscious level. It's as if you keep trying to resolve this wound by attracting emotionally distant partners and fighting for their love and affection. These kinds of relationships would also feel familiar to you; it's all you know, so it's not surprising that most of us end up in the same kind of relationship dynamics.

Grace makes such a powerful point here. Our adult relationships are not only attractive because they are unconsciously familiar—and we now know that the mind loves finding patterns like a heat seeking missile—but also because we seek to solve for a pain point, like a good emotional entrepreneur. We go from scenario to scenario attempting to rewrite our childhood story, with the wish for the happy ending, and the happy ending is where we are loved, cared for, protected, safe, stable, seen, and heard. This is the most noble story for any child, and it would embody a securely attached relationship with a parent.

The risk is that when we are in a toxic relationship, like the one with a narcissist, where the outcome is never secure attachment, we can get stuck in an obsessive loop to solve the story... but unbeknownst to us, we're in the wrong story with the wrong character. It never gets solved with the narcissist, full stop.

These patterns run really deep, and we remain unconscious of them until we begin doing the inner work. Over time, we become programmed and wired this way—our neural pathways reinforce these patterns, and we develop an energetic blueprint that subconsciously attracts us to partners who mirror the same dynamics. In a way, these relationships bring our wounds to the surface, giving us the opportunity to heal. But true freedom comes when we consciously recognize these patterns, do the inner work, and intentionally break the cycle.

When I started learning about the four types of attachment styles, I realized that I fell into the most extreme and challenging attachment style: disorganized/fearful avoidant. I couldn't deny it any longer as it perfectly described who I was in relationships and how I was feeling.

For years, during my relationships and after leaving the narcissist, I experienced a confusing mixture of wanting to love and connect with others, while having an extreme fear of intimacy simultaneously. As you can imagine, this type of attachment style makes it very difficult to develop healthy and secure relationships.

I never understood why I felt repulsed by decent guys who wanted an authentic and intimate relationship with me, but now everything started to make sense. Even though I craved true love and connection, subconsciously I knew that the narcissist couldn't give that to me, which was perfectly aligned with how I was, since I feared intimacy and vulnerability.

I realized that my mind was just trying to protect me from getting hurt, thus not allowing me to be true, authentic, and vulnerable in a relationship. But when you're not ready to show yourself as you really are with no masks, how can you expect someone to love you for who you really are? Of course, the narcissist was not the right person to try this out with. I realized that I needed to find a partner who made me feel safe to put my guard down and be vulnerable.

The unconscious conundrum here is that Grace's inherited relational pattern strangely felt "safe" in a disorganized, fear-ridden relationship because it's what she knew. Familiar—although destructive—can feel safe. So many people won't leave situations and people because the fear of the new is stronger than the fear of what is known. Herein lies the meaning of the "better the devil you know than the devil you don't" saying. A new type of attachment style, first, will not plug into the socket and, as she said, could feel repulsive, and second, may engender more fear because it is unknown and would require relational skills she had not developed yet.

Once I became aware of my attachment style, I realized that I needed to work on myself first before I could be able to build a healthy and secure relationship with someone else. This realization helped me understand that I needed to heal my own wounds and stop waiting for someone to come save me. It was time to start giving myself the love that I deeply desired in order to break this pattern of trying to get someone else to heal my pain.

Before I go on to explain how you can change your attachment style, let's have a look at the four different types of attachment styles as described by psychoanalyst John Bowlby and psychologist Mary Ainsworth.

The Four Attachment Styles

Secure Attachment Style

If as a child you perceived your parents as a secure base, and you felt comfortable being autonomous to explore the world independently, it's highly likely that you developed a secure attachment style. This means that romantic relationships in adulthood also feel safe and secure for you. People with secure attachment styles are able to feel connected, while still allowing themselves and their partners to move freely, and continue growing as individuals without being clingy in a relationship. Both partners in a secure relationship offer support to each other when feeling distressed, and they also seek each other for comfort when they feel troubled. So, everything is reciprocated rather than being on- sided. Their relationship tends to be honest, open, and equal, with both people feeling independent and loving toward each other.

People with a secure attachment style have healthy relationships where both partners can grow and thrive together. They understand how to merge together to form a stable ground. As a result, individuals with a secure attachment style feel more satisfied in their relationships. This doesn't mean that their relationships and dynamics are perfect. People with a secure attachment style also experience conflict and bad days, just like any other couple. But they are able to communicate effectively and solve problems rather than become defensive and attack their partners. Individuals who develop a secure attachment pattern are highly resilient, and they understand how to move past obstacles with great care and self-awareness.

Anxious Preoccupied Attachment Style

If, as a child, you experienced inconsistent and misattuned parenting, it's more likely that you develop an anxious attachment style. People with an anxious attachment style tend to approach relationships from a place of emotional hunger and feel desperate to form a bond with their partner. Individuals with this kind of attachment style unconsciously try to resolve the emotional neglect that they experienced in childhood, and expect their partner to rescue or complete them. However, they are not able to trust partners and feel safe with them. So they end up seeking a sense of safety and security by clinging to them. Unfortunately, this kind of behavior most often pushes their partner away from them.

Their behavior exacerbates their own fears. When they feel unsure of their partner's feelings and unsafe in their relationship, they become clingy, demanding, or possessive toward their partner. Most often, they also interpret independent actions by their partner as an affirmation of their fears. This kind of fear drives them to become even more clingy and suffocating, and they end up pushing their partner further away. As their partner pulls back, they strengthen their fear of being abandoned, and the emotional hunger is intensified. This scenario reaffirms that they were right about their fears, and as a result, they manifest their biggest fear of being abandoned into their reality.

Dismissive-Avoidant Attachment Style

If, during your childhood, your need for connection was disregarded, it's highly likely that you develop a dismissive avoidant attachment style. This means that you become emotionally distant and feel uncomfortable with intimate connections to protect yourself from being hurt. Most often, individuals with this type of attachment style seek isolation and feel that they cannot rely on anybody, so they end up parenting themselves. As adults, they come off as self-focused and may be overly focused on their basic needs and comforts. Every human being needs a connection with others, and believing that a human being can be fully independent is an illusion, as humans are social beings with a basic need for connection.

In heated or emotional situations, they are able to turn off their feelings instead of becoming reactive. If at any point their partner threatens to leave them, they have the ability to shut their emotions and pretend that they are indifferent. As a result, people with dismissive avoidant attachment styles have few intimate relationships and tend to deny the importance of loved ones in their life. In order to protect themselves, they developed a strong psychological defense and have the ability to detach from their partners. Having the space to grow individually when in a relationship is healthy. However, pushing your partner away to avoid being vulnerable indicates that you need to do the inner work so you can feel safe and secure in relationships.

Disorganized/Fearful Avoidant Attachment Style

Fearful-avoidant attachment style is the most extreme of the insecure attachment styles. If you identify with this kind of attachment style, keep in mind that you can still change it just like I did. If, as a child, you learned that the same person who is responsible for keeping you safe can also cause you emotional pain, even if unintentionally, you become scared of trusting that person with your feelings and vulnerabilities. In adulthood, you end up desiring love and connection while fearing intimacy and vulnerability at the same time. This can be very confusing and frustrating, as you feel like you have two strong forces pushing you and pulling you in opposite directions. As a result, you end up being distant from your romantic partner and hold back from building intimate and authentic relationships.

People who form this kind of attachment style alternate between two biological drives when it comes to emotional and intimate connections: the need to belong, love, and connect with others, and the need to survive and protect oneself. In romantic relationships, people with this type of attachment style feel scared and anxious when forming intimate relationships, and suffer from a negative self-image and damaging self-talk. They often feel intense loneliness, longing for genuine connection, but the stress and fear response makes them act erratically, driving away potential connection. Individuals with disorganized attachment styles pull away and tend to be emotionally distant to prevent themselves from being hurt and rejected.

They tend to see signs of rejection even when none are present in the relationship. Even if the potential partner may be expressing genuine interest, they might not trust that it is authentic, and their erratic behavior may cause the potential partner to lose interest. This further enforces the negative inner core beliefs; that he or she is unwanted and unlovable, leaving them feeling overwhelmed by their emotions. As a result, they face a constant inner battle between craving intimacy and resisting it at the same time. Their relationships often alternate between being clingy when they fear rejection and feeling trapped when they get too close. Individuals with disorganized attachment styles have a higher risk of ending up in toxic and dramatic relationships with many highs and lows.

They attempt to control their feelings to prevent causing drama but are unable to as their feelings are too overwhelming. As a result, they are overwhelmed by their reactions and often experience emotional storms. People with disorganized attachment styles end up perceiving relationships as dangerous because the person they seek safety from is the same person they fear getting close to. As a consequence, they have no organized strategy for getting their needs met by their partners.

Changing Your Attachment Style

Changing your attachment style is challenging and uncomfortable. When you invite awareness and you identify your attachment style, you can start becoming aware of the behaviors and patterns preventing you from building healthy relationships and developing an intimate emotional connection to others. Doing the inner work and nourishing yourself with self-love will help you heal your childhood wounds and slowly shift towards a secure attachment style and loving relationships. But to be able to have loving relationships, we first need to learn how to fall in love with ourselves.

At first, you might feel helpless against this deeply entwined attachment style because your brain has been wired and programmed that way. Awareness gives you the power to change, and practicing mindfulness can help you become self-aware and deepen the relationship with yourself. Realize that you are responsible for your own change and transformation. If you keep making the same choices and following the same patterns, you will get the same results and situations over and over again.

Be encouraged: Mindful awareness automatically changes the pattern. In a repeated science experiment, wherein most variables and processes stay the same, the mere changing of only one variable, changes the entire experiment. By becoming the mindful observer of your repetitive pattern, you have started the ball rolling in changing the pattern; you observing the pattern—or attachment style-is the new variable. Prior to that, it was unconsciously running. By adding the knowledge of the four attachment styles, you've now added another variable, new data, in addition to observing. See how the pattern (or experiment) is changing already?

Basically, if the pattern is one collapsed particle of the ever-changing waves of quantum possibilities, adding the possibilities of four attachment styles provides you with more possibilities. Imagine what happens when seeking more and more self-awareness, studying yourself, and adding more knowledge, like reading this book! You now have an entirely new experiment that lays down hope for new possibilities. My 4 P's may be helpful to memorize here: pause, power, possibility, and prowess. Pausing and observing gives you the power to decide a new response, which empowers you towards possibility (possibility is a future) and ultimately gives you prowess over your own life.

To unlearn bad habits in attachment, you need to be compassionate and patient with yourself because it takes time to heal and learn new ways of being. Learning how to make yourself feel safe, supported, and reassured is definitely a great start to healing.

If you have any of the attachment styles other than secure attachment, the act of being compassionate, patient, and loving to yourself automatically changes your attachment style, if we apply the framework of the scientific experiment. The pattern—let's say it's an entity in and of itself—begins to feel loved, understood, and safe; it doesn't care where that new data is coming from (you). It begins to form a new layer of neural pathways, and over time, this new mental model will scan and find securely attached experiences on its own. Isn't it beautiful that it's in your hands? You can provide your mental models, attachment style, and neural pathways a new self-love experience that will ultimately manifest in your external world.

Remember the neuroscientific phrase, "The more you fire, the more you wire." Isn't it beautiful that you don't have to outsource this experience of secure attachment to another, and can actually generate it yourself if you didn't receive it as a child? And worry not, slowly but surely, on its own, like a heat-seeking missile, it will recognize the familiar pattern in someone who will embody secure attachment for you. The old pattern will no longer match. This work is worthwhile for this alone! I posit that in finding securely attached friendships and communities, even if not romantic, we are helping that new attachment style to form and develop.

Trust that by being a part of self-healing communities like spiritual groups, psychotherapy groups, or 12-step programs, it "fires and wires" new ways of being and relating.

When you stop relying on other people to feel secure and loved, you realize that you have all the power in your hands. It is understandable that as a child, you depended on your parents or caregivers to feel safe and fulfill your needs. However, as an adult, it's dangerous and risky to depend on others to feel safe and secure. The outer world and the people in our lives are constantly changing, and it's easy to find yourself trapped in this loop where you keep trying to get others to make you feel safe, loved, and complete. To shift to a secure attachment style, you need to learn how to feel whole and complete by yourself; otherwise, it will be difficult to build healthy and secure relationships.

Working on changing your attachment style can be a solo journey. But since it can be quite challenging and you can easily fall back into old habits, I highly recommend that you seek support from professionals during this transformation. With appropriate therapy and support, it will be easier to learn new skills like recognizing, verbalizing, and communicating your thoughts and feelings. Therapy can also help you and support you when testing the waters in future relationships. When working with a professional, you can learn how to feel safe communicating your needs and emotions instead of making premature assumptions that lead to acting out insecure attachment styles.

Rephrasing internal negative self-talk is also a powerful tool that will help you with your transformation. The mind can sabotage new relationships out of fear and self-protection. If one believes that he or she is unlovable, this will come out in the relationship, and no matter what your partner does, your actions will be self-destructive and can lead to pushing your partner away. Choosing a kind, reliable, and honest partner will definitely help you shift toward a healthy attachment style. You need to feel safe in the relationship so you can feel like you can rely on and trust your partner. Otherwise, if you choose toxic partners, the dynamics of your relationship will reaffirm your beliefs and ideas about a relationship, and will make it impossible for you to adopt a secure attachment style. It's like you're throwing vinegar on a wound that's trying to heal.

With time, practice, and awareness, it gets easier to make conscious choices. Eventually, you will realize that you are making minimal effort to hold yourself against any impulsive reactions that would cause unnecessary turbulence in your relationships. The new you becomes your true nature, and looking back at who you were, you barely recognize yourself. Give credit to yourself as you are progressing, it will help you stay motivated and empowered to keep moving forward until the unhealthy behavioral patterns and tendencies dissolve.

Building a relationship based on trust, authentic love, and acceptance doesn't mean that everything will always be perfect. But it will surely help you communicate your needs and resolve conflicts with less drama. The effort and dedication required to make these changes are truly worth it as you set yourself free from the emotional baggage you have been carrying since you were a child.

Shifting to a secure attachment style will help you attract emotionally available men who are ready to love you and accept you for who you are. They treat you with respect, and support you to help you grow and thrive in your life. But first, you need to become that person who attracts those kinds of men.

And that involves:

- Respecting yourself
- Setting boundaries
- Accepting who you are
- Communicating your needs and emotions
- Being able to enjoy your own company
- Supporting yourself to grow and thrive
- Being authentic with yourself and others
- Knowing who you are, what you want, and what you don't want

INSIGHTFUL LESSON: Self-love gives you freedom. Fear doesn't permanently leave you, but you will find the strength within you to move mountains. Self-love heals everything.

Inner Child Healing Exercise

This exercise is all about connecting with your inner child and helping your inner child feel safe. By parenting ourselves and providing our inner child with unconditional love and the security that we need helps us heal our unresolved wounds:

Step 1: Find a quiet space somewhere where you won't be disturbed. Take a comfortable position and close your eyes. Make sure you are feeling supported and grounded in your chair or lying down.

Step 2: Take five deep, mindful breaths, focusing your attention on your breaths. Notice the air coming in through your nose as you inhale, filling up your stomach. Notice how your tummy goes down as you exhale and you release the air.

Step 3: With your eyes closed, bring up a memory in your mind's eye of when you were a kid and you felt like you were scared or in need of love and protection. See yourself as a kid as vividly and clearly as possible.

Step 4: Go over to your inner child in the memory and give your inner child a deep, loving hug. Tell your inner child and reassure her that you are there for her now and that you will always protect her. Promise her that you will be more present with her and that you will start paying attention to her needs. Help her feel reassured that she is safe, loved, and secure with you.

Step 5: When you feel ready, you can let your inner child go and come back to the present moment. You might feel the need to cry or a strong sense of compassion for your inner child. This is completely natural, and if you feel the need to cry, allow your emotions to surface and leave your body. Always keep in mind that this feeling is only temporary, and it too shall pass.

Step 6: When you feel like you have released as much as you could, close your eyes once again and take 3 deep mindful breaths. Bring up a memory in your mind's eye when you were feeling happy and joyful as a child. Focus on how you were feeling and what you were doing. Allow yourself to experience the playfulness of your inner child and bring it back with you to the present moment.

Step 7: Before you carry on with your day, set your intention to be more connected with your inner child and nurture her needs. Provide her with love, safety, and compassion, and listen to what she needs.

Repeat this exercise whenever you need to nurture and reassure your inner child to heal the unresolved wounds. It's okay if you need to do it more than once. Traumas and emotional pain take time and lots of self-love and compassion to heal.

I absolutely adore all of Grace's suggested exercises. They are so complete and on point. I would add very little. My suggestions are more body-based and visceral, as I've discovered through my own journey and holistic approach. Ensuring the body absorbs new information in a safe manner is central to healing, since it was the site where much of the injury was also recorded. Also in my approach is making the disclaimer that "weird is ok" and what I mean by this is that if you are a trauma survivor, suffer from high anxiety, panic attacks, or ADHD, there are things that may feel relieving or soothing to your inner child that may look or feel weird.

For example, I encourage my trauma folks to swaddle themselves with body pillows on each side when doing inner child work. Another possibility is curl up under a soft blanket or a weighted blanket—on the floor is best for grounding—swaddled by pillows, so that the inner child feels surrounded in a safe embrace, per se, and metaphorically tucked in, an experience that did not likely happen as a child. I also suggest adding beautiful, tender, and angelic music—lullabies, even—to create a full experience of soothing the inner child. Lullabies or tender music create an innocent and safe environment. In essence, allow your whole body to feel child-like in whatever way that means.

Journal Prompts

What emotional needs are you still trying to fulfill by others?

What kind of needs are not being met and fulfilled in your relationship/previous relationships?

How does this make you feel?

Recall a memory from your childhood when you were trying to get your needs met by your parents or caregivers. What did you do?

What similarities can you see between how you felt back then and now in your relationship?

What changes do you need to make to start getting your emotional needs met in a healthy way?

What kind of qualities does a person need to have to meet your emotional needs in your relationship in a healthy way?

I'm big on daily and weekly practices. In fact, when people seek to work with me, I have added a question to my interview process asking whether they participate in any holistic practices, like the ones Grace describes. Weekly or bi-monthly psychotherapy sessions will not be enough to make healing changes in one's life. In fact, I believe that psychotherapy, mentoring, or coaching sessions are a "practice" of self-observation and self-inquiry. Our lives need to be threaded together by well-being exercises that include silence, stillness, movement, joy, writing, reading, and communing.

In my monthly spiritual roundtable, Wealth from Within, we call them "RICHuals," or practices that make our life feel more abundant and prosperous. There are so many things that fit into these categories...so many! The idea here is living the intentional life that re-directs towards healing and from trauma surviving into trauma rising. This is what I describe as the "Heaven on Earth" life, which is replete with self-exploration, self-knowledge, cultivating secure attachment bonds, healing the inner child, and a calm central nervous system.

Part IV

Recovering From Narcissistic Abuse

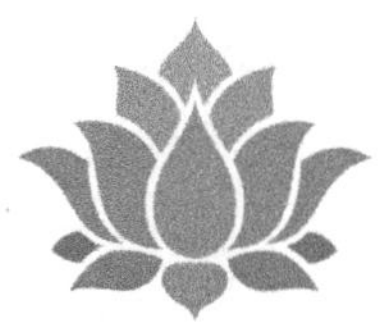

WELL DONE, WARRIOR. IF you've made it this far, it shows real commitment. It doesn't matter how long it takes you. It doesn't matter how many times you fall back. What matters is that you're here doing the inner work, becoming more mindful, and learning to recognize the narcissist's tactics, your wounds, and your patterns.

This final part of the book is a step-by-step guide to support your recovery from narcissistic abuse. Of course, healing isn't linear. It takes time, patience, and looks different for everyone. But this is your starting point.

As you grow more mindful, you begin to awaken to a deeper part of yourself. You create space within. You start receiving insights that once seemed out of reach. And as your self-awareness expands, so does your sense of free will.

Without mindfulness, we're likely to repeat the same patterns, not because we want to, but because our choices are still being driven by wounds and unconscious programming.

Practices like meditation, psychotherapy, dreamwork, walking meditation, yoga, ecstatic dance, sound healing, and other somatic tools have all played a crucial role in my journey. They've helped me reconnect with my inner strength, my inner light, and with a higher power that carried me through even the darkest times, when I had no idea how I'd keep going.

In the chaos of daily life, we tend to neglect the part of us that longs for spiritual nourishment. But we need it. Whether it comes through art, music, movement, nature, or something else entirely, nurturing the spiritual self is essential.

It's how we find our light. And it's that light that guides us from the darkest abyss to a place of peace and possibility on the other side of the journey.

May these chapters, and my personal experience with mindfulness and spirituality, awaken your inner flame just as mine was once awakened by my own guides and mentors on this journey.

Chapter 13

Acknowledging What Happened

RECOVERING FROM NARCISSISTIC ABUSE is a pain in the ass, but going through it is way worse. So when you embark on the path of healing, remind yourself that it can only get better from here. I'm not going to lie to you or sugarcoat it; this process takes time, and it is not the same for everyone. It could take months or even years. In my case, I needed years of inner work, and I focused on nobody else but myself.

What a powerful way to start this chapter and this healing journey, facing the demon square in the eye. Let's discuss this thoroughly from multiple angles.

I deem it essential to be completely alone for a period of time to recover from narcissistic abuse. I liken it to sobriety or a detoxification. We must get as close to our original baseline as we possibly can. We must go in and reprogram our neural pathways with repetitive new thinking and feeling—carefully and deliberately chosen by us—in order to regain trust in our ability to choose. We must completely reformat the way we engage, relate, and love.

Relational sobriety, in itself, allows for a non-judgmental space to examine the psychological clutter within us and undergo the process of purging and organizing. We get to re-discover ourselves without the hating and critical lens of the narcissist, who intentionally shatters our sense of self. We have the time to put back those identity puzzle pieces and add new ones. Ultimately, at the end of this journey, the treasure at the base of the rainbow is that we get to trust ourselves anew. TRUST is the ultimate intra-relational and inter-relational treasure. My heart feels full writing this. You get the gift of trusting yourself.

So yes, like a food or allergy detox, after a time spent alone in self-healing and self-exploration, start considering what you can add back by how it makes you feel. Review your friendships, family members, and even colleagues, and decide who is allowed back. Base this welcoming on how you feel—is it disruptive? Is it anxiety-provoking? Do you feel seen, supported, and understood? Are you playful? What does your inner being say about this relationship? Reflect on whether you are having a PTSD flare-up around this person, or if you are consistently disrupted by how they are. Don't worry, let's be gentle...you don't have to have it all figured out. After spending time in some relational sobriety, your soul-body will help inform you.

When I was still with him, I had already started taking the necessary steps to grow and discover myself on a deeper level. Strengthening my sense of self-reliance and autonomy empowered me to build up the courage to leave him. I made many mistakes along the way, but it didn't matter as long as I was learning from them and becoming a better version of myself.

Looking back on my relationship, I didn't realize how toxic and abusive it was until things started to really heat up and get out of hand. When you are exposed to abusive behavior on a daily basis, it's easy to end up normalizing the abuse as it becomes your everyday life. Through gaslighting, he made me believe that his toxic behavior was normal.

As the abuse continued, I became more powerless and dependent on his validation. He always denied that he mistreated me in any way, and he accused me of being too sensitive. Eventually, I ended up questioning myself, and I started thinking that perhaps he was right, I was too sensitive, and I was exaggerating. I found myself always justifying his abuse, and I refused to acknowledge what was really happening, even when others pointed it out. Instead of acknowledging the abuse and manipulation, I was entirely focused on being good enough for him.

Letting go of this need to be validated and acknowledging that I was a victim of narcissistic abuse, helped me make sense out of things, and I realized that I was not crazy. A part of me felt ashamed for what happened, and I was angry at myself for being naive and for letting someone take advantage of me and manipulate me. Understanding the psychology behind narcissistic abuse helped me realize that everyone could fall for their games, no matter how smart you are or what status you hold in society.

This is a moment of choice between hard choices:

1) You can feel alone, defeated, and demeaned inside the relationship, or you can feel alone, scared, yet open to starting anew outside of the relationship.

2) You can face the external bully on a daily basis, exhaust yourself, and not get anywhere, in fact, go backwards, and become smaller, even invisible or you can face your internal bullies—the low self-worth, self-esteem, negative self-talk—and have a chance of transmuting them and transforming yourself.

3) You can stay with the narcissist. You can always stay. This is your sovereign choice, as long as it is conscious, it is yours. That's the whole impetus behind all self-reflection, healing, and consciousness raising:

we get to be the sovereign choosers of our life experience. Recognize that staying means self-mutilation via an external source. We don't recommend this option at all. We recommend the exact opposite. Do the hard work of leaving and choosing you. I find it important to offer staying as a choice because you must see it as an option amongst others and compare.

All are hard, period. The prognosis is what makes them different: some lead to hope and evolution, and other to despair and regression.

Once you acknowledge what you have experienced, you start making sense and finding answers to your questions. Even though it's extremely painful, it gives you a sense of relief, especially after having your feelings denied by the narcissist. Once we become aware of something, we can have a clearer look at what's happening and see how we can find a way out of the situation we find ourselves in.

A note: Even if you are relationally sober—and remember, the narcissist can be a lover, a family member, a parent, a child, a boss, a culture (yes, a narcissistic culture!)—and have chosen to be alone, you don't have to do the process alone. Sources like this book, like Grace, who is a coach specialized in this topic, support groups, 12-step groups, and endless internet conversations about the topic, are a way to feel supported and swaddled through what I call "the bridge and tunnel work." Sometimes it feels like we are crawling our way to the light, but even so, crawl forward and know that there are survivors in front of you, beside you, and behind you. You are not alone, so don't do it alone. In fact, that's the first step in recovering from the narcissist who isolated you in the first place. Find the persons, places, or things where you feel flanked by others.

Acknowledging what happened is the first step that will allow you to start taking action to change your life. From that point onward, you can transform yourself from a victim of narcissistic abuse into an empowered warrior who has taken control of their life and rewritten their story.

Journal Prompts

#1. How are you feeling today? What makes you feel this way?

#2. What areas of your life are causing you the most emotional pain?

#3. What lessons have you learned from this challenging and painful experience?

#4. What steps and actions can you take to improve your situation and protect yourself?

#5. What painful experience or memory are you ready to release today?

An exercise I would add here is my "saying yes" meditation, in this case, this is done in order to arrive at a confident, self-validating truth. Start your time by closing your eyes and placing a hand over where you are having a feeling. Ask yourself what you are feeling, maybe something like, "What am I longing for, wishing, or wanting from the narcissist?" When the answer "pops," validate it. For example, "I need safe loving" or "I need to feel seen and cared for" or "I long to be married and have my own children" or "I crave consistency."...then say to yourself and to your inner child, "Of course I do."

Even when your longings feel desperate and can therefore be buried by shame, allow them to come up by saying yes to them. Place your hand over where you feel it and say yessss, over and over, while breathing out. You may have a desperate longing to feel understood, to feel held, to feel excited for, etc. Say yes to it and then say, "Of course you do." These are basic human needs. Basic human needs. These feelings are the ingredients to secure attachment, and the level at which you long for them—maybe desperately—is the level at which you did not receive them. Validate these basic human needs and desires by saying yes to them and then by saying, "Of course, sweet one, of course."

Release your emotional pain through healthy channels and exercises like the one described at the end of Chapter 2.

Here are some other tips that you can use to release your emotional pain:

- Crying*
- Body movement
- Meditation
- Yoga
- Physical exercise
- Painting/Art
- Dancing
- Singing
- Journaling

**Crying is a way of releasing your pain out of your body and psyche. Just make sure that you don't get stuck there too long, and follow it up by doing something that raises your vibration and makes you feel joyful.*

Chapter 14

Understanding Trauma Bonding

WHEN YOU'RE IN A relationship with a narcissist, you think that you're madly and deeply in love with the person. You feel like you're addicted. It feels like you are being dragged by an invisible force pulling you towards him. I tried to resist my desperate need for his attention and validation. I was completely unaware of what was really going on, and I had mistaken this desperate need for validation for love.

I find the addictive framework applicable and helpful in understanding the relationship with the narcissist because there is so much overlap. It is also a framework that allows for a more "technical" approach to recovery, versus the belief that it is a redeemable relationship for which to stay; fighting for love versus fighting to free yourself from an addiction are two separate paradigms.

In SLAA—Sex and Love Addicts Anonymous—the premise is that you have a relationship wherein both partners are locked into a codependent relationship with a shared history of abandonment, neglect, and/or traumatic event(s). This ruptured childhood attachment style has laid the foundation for seeking relationships as the "cure-all" for this endless attachment longing. Maybe this lover will fill the desperate longing for love never filled as a child? The relationship is based on a symbiotic and interlocked cycle of converging, fighting, abandoning, and returning with the hopes of restoring the original romance (chasing the original high), followed by a devolving pattern of more despair, which fuels and reinforces the cycle even more. Both players are protagonists and co-dependent in the addictive pattern.

Naturally, there are more details to this relational addiction, but for the purpose of this section, it's useful to see the correlation from an aerial perspective, particularly to note that "it takes two to tango" in spite of it seeming that the narcissist is in control of everything. It's quite the contrary, as the narcissist cannot live without the victim's (wounded Empath) supply. Remember, the victim/wounded Empath/you can not only live without the narcissist, but you can shine in your own right. The narcissist cannot.

During one particular healing session, my healer asked me whether I believed that it was really love that I felt for this person. I was confused and I didn't really understand what he meant. I assured him that it was indeed love. He explained to me that love doesn't involve emotional and verbal abuse, and that it doesn't involve suffering. When he started going deeper into his interpretation of what love is, I realized that I didn't know the meaning and the feeling of love at all. When, later on in life, I experienced what love really felt like, I realized how wrong I was.

Trauma bonding is the real reason why you feel so addicted to the narcissist and crave him like a drug. If you take a look at your relationship, you will realize that the narcissist plays a very subtle, yet powerful and effective emotional mind game. They alternate back and forth between periods of manipulation, gaslighting, and abuse, and periods of love bombing where they get your hopes up and make you feel like you're the most special person in the world. According to the article on Psych Central (2019), narcissists employ trauma bonding and intermittent reinforcement to create an addiction to them, which may explain why abuse survivors stay ("Narcissists Use Trauma Bonding and Intermittent Reinforcement").

Intermittent positive reinforcement leaves you feeling confused and craving the return of those euphoric good moments. Every time the narcissist starts making you feel good again in the relationship, your brain releases chemicals such as oxytocin and dopamine, which make you feel good and can be addictive. These chemicals are also released in the brain when people make use of substances like opiates, alcohol, nicotine, amphetamines, and cocaine. That's how potent and addictive narcissists can be.

Indeed, intermittent reinforcement or that "rollercoaster" feeling is a key component to the pleasure factor in an addictive relationship. It feels exciting, dramatic, and close to the edge. I submit that when we have had a childhood of neglect or trauma, we know exactly what it's like to feel so close to the edge that we don't know what it's like to live in the land of peace, safety, and stability. We've always been hanging out near the cliff, on the verge of the abyss: the abyss of abuse, the abyss of loneliness, the abyss of invisibility, the abyss of chaos.

Two things are perpetuated with the addictive narcissist relationship, then: 1) the familiarity of the roller coaster life, with intermittent attention; and 2) the activation of the childhood neural pathway of what I call "edge-of-cliff" living. I find this doesn't just relate to childhood experiences of trauma, but of adult experiences of trauma as well, where coming back from psychic or physical near-death experiences feels nearly impossible, uncomfortable, and/or boring.

Because the nature of secure attachment or a healthy relationship requires safety, stability, and consistency, securely attached relationships or "normal life" can first be experienced as boring to those who are recovering from an addiction or C-PTSD. Know that this is a common stage at the start of recovery. While the urge to return to that rollercoaster ride of intermittent highs can feel quite compelling, I recommend a holistic approach to recovery—one where your mind, body, heart, and spirit have the time to absorb new information and acclimate to a new pattern of existence.

As you can see, trauma bonding makes it very hard for the victims to leave the relationship. It would be much easier to leave someone who was always making you feel miserable. But with a narcissist, it feels like you're on an emotional roller coaster with the highs and lows. During that period of rejection, you long for positive reinforcement to relieve the emotional suffering and feel good about yourself, until you are rejected once again. It's a vicious cycle that keeps you trapped in the relationship.

A loving relationship doesn't involve being mistreated, given the silent treatment, and being rejected just because your partner is in a bad mood or something bad happened to them during the day. When you develop trauma bonding, you willingly forgive your narcissist for just about anything. You start making excuses for their abusive behavior and justify it by saying that they had a bad day or that they're going through a rough time. When I started getting back to my senses, I understood that just because someone is going through a rough period doesn't mean that it's okay to engage in abusive behavior. Ask yourself, is that how you treat your narcissist when you're having a bad day? Any kind of abusive behavior is completely unacceptable, no matter what the circumstances are. Let's face it, we all face different challenges and situations in life, and how we react to them reflects the kind of person we are.

Trauma bonds are very powerful and can last from several months up to a few years. For some people, it might not fade away completely and can take longer to fully recover. The more time you spend in the relationship, the longer the trauma bond might last.

Because of my multicultural and multilingual background, I find it easy and helpful to approach trauma bonding as a culture and a language. It is a habitual way we live with each other and talk about life. I slightly joke and emphasize the example we often use in Spanish to greet each other: "Como estás?" (How are you?) and the response, "Acá, siempre en la lucha" (Here, always in the struggle). This is one of many greetings, of course, but it's a very common one.

Furthermore, trauma bonding is actually ingrained in certain cultures, and it is, in truth, how people speak and connect with each other. I want to make this point for those of you who are in cultural contexts where narcissism and trauma bonding are a way of life. There are some of you who will read this book and may despair at realizing that you are surrounded by a system of beliefs and relational engagements that are deeply rooted in narcissistic abuse and its concentric circles of accompanying trauma. You may be surrounded by victims of ancestral and current narcissistic wounding, and thus, trauma bonding amongst the victims marked by a perpetual grieving over the circumstances, an acceptance of this way of life, and a pessimism or criticism about any other way of life, leaves you feeling like there is no way out.

There is, there is, there is a way out! If this book is in your hands, you are divinely meant to find another way and to search for your healing! Know that there is a world beyond what you're experiencing—even if your grandparents, parents, aunties, uncles, and best friends—are all in the same inherited system and are going through the same things, even if they say, "That's our way of life" or "It is what it is" or "Don't abandon your family, culture, or religion." Know at your very core, this is not the way for any human.

Yes, to subjugate, enslave, and demean, and yes, to repeatedly enact the victim-aggressor-savior paradigm has been a part of human history; it fills most of our religious texts and history books. It is not, however, the original human story of being divinely created, loved, and created for love. We are all biologically born with empathic hearts and the adaptive mammalian ability to care for and protect one another. Protecting and caring for one another has kept us alive as a species, as we see by the creation of hospitals, shelters, support groups, sanctuaries, activism, psychologies, books...books like this one. We are compelled, inspired, encouraged, motivated, and called to care and help each other, and this is the very reason we have not gone extinct as a species.

Know that there is a door that opens to other cultures, languages, and chosen families that bond around trauma rising and empathic care, rather than trauma bonding and victim-aggressor relating. Notice that you are here, now.

Let's have a look at some of the major signs that you have developed trauma bonding with the narcissist.

Your Relationship Feels Toxic

This is pretty obvious, right? If you're reading this book, it means that you're very well aware that your relationship is toxic and that there's something very wrong with your relationship dynamics. If you find yourself feeling anxious after a few weeks without conflict in the relationship, it's because you know that your good moments never last for too long. So, you subconsciously start thinking about when the next storm will hit. Do you really want your whole life to be like this?

Consider that the feeling of "waiting for the other shoe to drop" is an internal program that is running because of a childhood experience that precedes your current adult relationship. There are a few options when you have the constant dread that "something bad is going to happen, even when it all seems good." Grace is right in pointing to the likelihood that this current relationship is poisoned with this foreboding. However, I'd like to suggest that it may come from a prior time, and you may be the "carrier" of the feeling.

This internal program (schema, neural pathway, mental model, psychological pattern, etc.) can come from the volatile moods of an alcoholic, abusive, and/or bipolar caregiver, wherein it was common for things to be good in one moment and change drastically in another. It can also come from experiences of feeling financially safe and then having the electricity cut off or being evicted. These internal formulas look like happy=sad, safe=dread, love=loss, and so on.

The metaphor of living close to the cliff or the edge infuses the good moments with a dark, warning cloud of doom. Whether it comes from the current relationship or from your past—very likely from both, given that the mind navigates towards patterns—it is paramount that this program be observed and transmuted into love can equal love, happy can equal happy, love can equal safe, and good can equal better. Remember, it's in doing the internal work that our external world shifts, to include all sorts of beautiful characters and experiences.

You Feel Powerless and Submissive

If you feel controlled by your partner in any way, it's a form of manipulation. Manipulation doesn't necessarily involve direct threats. It is often subtle and indirect, yet still highly effective. For example, if the narcissist throws a tantrum every time you don't submit to their needs, you start noticing the pattern, even if they claim to be arguing with you about something completely unrelated. In your heart, you know the real reason why he's throwing the tantrum, even though you cannot explain it. If you find yourself being submissive to avoid big fights or negative behaviors from your partner, it's a sign of power imbalance and abuse. Do you want to continue living in fear with this person?

I include manipulation as a form of emotional molestation, the behavior I coined and described earlier that is particularly injurious to children and Empaths because they are highly sensitive and are prone—if not hardwired—to harmonize environments where there is tension or conflict. The wounded Empath or the child may, over time, become more and more silent and make themselves "invisible" in order to placate the abusive, explosive, and even complaining narcissist as a way to create homeostasis.

Britannica defines homeostasis as "any self-regulating process by which an organism tends to maintain stability while adjusting to conditions that are best for its survival." Examples are becoming more and more quiet or hidden vis-à-vis the narcissistic explosions or becoming the fixer/savior to soothe the complaining or suffering parent. We discussed the zombie-like state, and when I teach about wounded Empaths, I call it the disappearing Empath, as they leave their bodies until they have no personality left. This is how Grace found herself at the start of her healing journey, unable to even identify what she liked on Netflix.

You've Left Before But You Keep Going Back

Even though logically it doesn't make sense, you feel like no matter what happens, you'll always end up going back to him. Your attempts to set boundaries have been flushed down the drain. You fear being without them, as you are scared that you will become a nobody without the narcissist. You've lost your ability to feel good about yourself without their validation and approval. It might feel safer to stay in an abusive relationship instead of being alone due to the intense fear of abandonment. Do you really think that being with your own company is worse than being with a narcissist?

The answer to this for many has been, "Yes, my own company is worse, and my panic to be alone feels insurmountable" when they first start to disengage from the narcissist. A few words of hope: remember that there are millions of alcoholics and addicts who felt the same way each time they relapsed; remember that it is the syndrome of "the evil I know is better than anything I don't know," and that syndrome can be overcome. There exists a world of healing, with structure, steps, and success rates for those who have left, like Grace. No matter where you are, there is a well-paved way of people who have found themselves on the other side.

There Are Good Moments But Too Many Bad Ones

Do you find yourself reminiscing about the good moments and asking yourself why it cannot be like that forever? If the bad moments outweigh the good ones, then what's the point of being together? It can be tempting to just forget everything bad that happened and get lost in the love bombing period once your abuser starts using their charm again. But is it worth it knowing that it's just a matter of time until they break you again?

A good exercise for those moments of reminiscing about the good times is to write them down, yes, alongside the horrible memories. Give the horrible ones more detail, because in those moments when the narcissist comes back strong or appears to be suffering or punishes you by withholding love, it's very easy for your mind to resort to the good memories. This occurs especially with those who are empathic, as they naturally gravitate towards seeing the good in people and understand their suffering deeply within themselves.

If in those moments you can look at several journal entries where you see, in detail, the horrible ways you were spoken to, the names you were called, the continuous and consistent ways you were mistreated, it helps. It helps to have conviction, even as the impulse may be to return.

Please remember that I am speaking not only about a lover here, but I am also speaking about a parent, a friend, a boss, or even an adult addicted child. The volatile and destructive cycles are similar for each. The Empath will feel like they are going against their very nature to reject the narcissist, and they will feel like they are wounding another human. The child will feel like they are hurting a caregiver or protector, and that they won't survive. These are all natural, caring, human responses, but in drastically sadistic situations. Remind yourself by writing those memories down.

You Justify Your Partner's Behavior

If you find yourself justifying why your partner is mistreating you, it's a big sign of trauma bonding. Just because someone had a bad day at work or is going through a rough period does not mean it's okay to accept abusive and manipulative behavior. Our actions and reactions toward our human experience define who we are. Everyone goes through difficult moments in their lives, but how you handle them defines who you are and what kind of personality you have. Even if your partner had a traumatic past, it doesn't make it okay to accept their abusive behavior. Do you really think abusive behavior is acceptable for any reason? Why?

This is written and asked beautifully here. I find it helpful to distill these behaviors to "human to human" behaviors because when it is someone to whom you are biologically connected or someone with whom you fell in love, it is easier to enable bad behavior because you understand them. Tolerance is extended because you know them. When we distill it to the "human to human" framework, it may be easier to objectively see that any human treating another abusively is not acceptable.

I like to give examples such as: 'Would you accept rage from someone standing in front of you in line because they had a bad day?' or, 'Would you accept a teacher screaming or punishing your child because they were in a mood?' 'Would you accept abuse or aggression from someone in an elevator because they were drunk?'

Would you accept these behaviors from any other human you don't know? No matter the biological connection, the age, the race, the ethnicity, the religion, the tradition, when you drop the "human to human" filter on it, what is your perspective? This is not an easy question to ask and look at because you may be in a family structure where it is normal for the parent to go off at the dinner table, where the father is never questioned, or where abusive beatings are part of how things have been done. In spite of this, you can dig deep and say to yourself, "From human to human, this is not ok and I now choose to do this differently." That internal decision begins reversing the momentum.

You Are Scared to Tell Your Friends & Family

You might feel scared or ashamed to share your concerns and anxieties with your friends and family. The narcissist might warn you not to tell anyone about your private life together. You might also try to protect their reputation, so you find yourself hiding the truth to protect their image. If nothing was wrong in the relationship, why would you be scared of telling the truth? Why do you want to protect their reputation more than yourself?

Twelve-step programs have a very powerful adage: you are as sick as your secrets. The recovery journey highly emphasizes bringing secrets to the light in order to have a full recovery because addictions are generally kept hidden. As secrets remain in the dark corners, they fester, rot, and can get very stinky for generations to come. I would add that bringing our shame into the light is the start of the light shining through the wound.

In my communities and in my own healing journey, I call these "shame shares." Once a shame is shared—as torturous as it may feel in the moment and even in the moments following the share—something miraculous happens because it lightens the weight of carrying the secret, and it generally finds sanctuary in others who have the same secrets. In group psychotherapy, this is called "universality," a unifying and empowering group principle. Safe sharing in a group has miraculous healing powers. Find a group. There are many and they are free.

Feeling Obliged or Indebted

Narcissists make you feel like you owe them and that you're indebted to them. This is a form of manipulation and abuse of power. They do it intentionally and consistently to make you feel bad, so you constantly try to make it up to them. Did you ever stop to think about how much they owe you for your patience, kindness, generosity, forgiveness, and never- ending list of good gestures as you succumb to their selfish egoic needs? Do you want to be in a relationship where you are always made to feel inferior? Wouldn't it be more enjoyable to be in a relationship where there is equal reciprocation of giving and receiving?

Grace has said it all very clearly here. Beholdenness is a common narcissistic tactic. I'd like to underscore that many narcissistic parents and cultures do this. You must "pay the price" for what they gave you, even when you did not give birth to yourself. I deem it cruel to make a child feel indebted to what a parent provides for them; this indebtedness is the root of profound future issues of low self-worth, low self-esteem, money issues, and relational issues, such as falling for abusive partners. It relegates the child to "working" for the parents' love, earning what they receive, rather than receiving it as a natural-born-right between mature, adult caregivers and children. Notice the relationships that are based on feelings of obligation rather than a loving desire to give, share, care, and protect each other reciprocally.

Isolating Yourself

When you're going through an extreme amount of stress, anxiety, and emotional turbulence, you might isolate yourself as you feel scared and completely exhausted. Your family and friends might be arguing with you to leave your abuser. And you end up avoiding them or distancing yourself from people trying to help you, and you feel like no one understands you. The narcissist might also try to isolate you from everyone to make you more powerless and easier to manipulate. Surrounding yourself with people who truly love you and care about you will help you and support you as you get out of this situation. Why would you want to spend more time with someone who crushes your soul instead of people who are trying to help you get better?

These are all signs of trauma bonding, and becoming aware of them will help you make sense of what seems to be illogical behavior. Be compassionate with yourself, as what's happening is not your fault. It's a psychological addiction created by the narcissist. Just like I was able to break free from the trauma bond, you too can be free of this nightmare.

In the next chapter, we will discuss how you can break free from the trauma bond so you can reclaim your life and transform into your most beautiful, authentic, and powerful self.

Yes, this is a psychological addiction created by the narcissist, and I will add, a possible psychological mental model rooted in childhood familial, cultural, and ethnic experiences that creates a match for the narcissist. When healing and with much effort, this match changes naturally through the transmuting of the original pattern recognition.

Chapter 15

Breaking Free from the Trauma Bond

GOING THROUGH ANY KIND of breakup is painful, unpleasant, and can be quite messy until you readjust yourself and adapt to your new lifestyle. However, breaking up with a narcissist is a completely different ball game.

As explained in the previous chapter, trauma bonding makes it harder to let go of narcissists, even though they're literally the source of your emotional pain and trauma. Even though you can start working on the relationship with yourself to strengthen yourself and prepare to leave the narcissist, it's highly unlikely that you will break free from the trauma bond while you're still in the relationship or in contact with the narcissist.

Grace is so right when she describes how hard it is to be free from the narcissist for several reasons: if you have not identified your own addiction to the relationship you will likely return for the fix, like a relapse; the narcissist will usually come back strong or act like everything's back to normal (very common with narcissistic parents); and, you will have to confront the fear of being alone or the perpetual fear that you will not be loved by anyone else, like you weren't as a child. Most psychologists who work with narcissistic abuse recommend no contact because the pattern is so insidious, vicious, and self-fulfilling.

Trying to stop all contact with a narcissist feels like you are coming off a drug. This usually pushes people to fall back into the relationship as they feel powerless against their cravings and give in to their impulses. Returning to your abuser is extremely dangerous as this continues to damage your self-esteem, strengthens the trauma bond, and provides the narcissist with narcissistic supply.

It is also very dangerous because it gives the narcissist the misguided message that you will tolerate the abuse, and in fact, you came back for it. It underscores that you cannot live without them, and once you sign off on being dependent on them by coming back, the levels of abuse, whether physical or psychological, increase as par for the course. It behooves us to underscore even more strongly that when you leave, find immediate support (plan this before leaving). Even if you go back, know that you can leave and start over again. That is the promise of 12-step groups: no matter how many relapses, you can always start over, one day at a time.

When you decide to end the relationship and stop all contact with the narcissist, you need to make peace with the fact that you will not feel very good for a while. It's common to experience feelings of withdrawal and grief, but it's the only way you can free yourself from this nightmare and heal your emotional trauma.

Withdrawal symptoms is the perfect phrase for what to expect. In the Dynamic Meditation Method—my emotional calibrating modality—I use the phrase "your CNS is your CVS," and what that means is that your thoughts and their accompanying feelings have a direct impact on your central nervous system and serve as a literal pharmacy inside the body.

In toxic and dysfunctional relationships and families, our central nervous system has become addicted to a memorized way of responding to our external world, and we flood our system with cortisol showers stemming from volatility and deep feelings of longing and lack. It takes a while to detox from these automatic feelings and their ensuing chemical releases into the body. The good news is that just as our thoughts and feelings can release negative chemical waterfalls into our central nervous system, so it can release soothing and healing chemicals such as oxytocin, the love and trust hormone. Your CNS is your CVS. You will withdraw from the negative and can transition into the positive.

This can be a difficult journey, so surrounding yourself with friends and family to help you work through a difficult breakup is extremely helpful. Don't feel ashamed or scared to ask for help, what happened is not your fault, even if you might feel responsible for everything that you went through. Keep in mind that you have been conditioned to feel responsible for everything that goes wrong by the narcissist, but that doesn't make it true. Focus on nurturing the relationship with yourself and learn how to start loving yourself and treating yourself with respect. Practice setting boundaries so you start protecting yourself from any kind of abuse and manipulation.

Each time I left the narcissist, it felt really scary, as I always thought it was going to be the last time we contacted each other. To my surprise, he always came back trying to lure me in to meet him once again. There were times when I fell for my impulses and contacted him myself, but in the end, I had to be the one to end the relationship and all kinds of communication channels for good. So, when you decide to leave the narcissist, there's a huge chance that they will come back. It might be after a few weeks, months, or even years.

Indeed, remember that it's the narcissist who can't live without your supply. Imagine if you didn't have the abandonment wounds and the low self-worth that colluded with their threats of being nothing without them, you would have seen straight through their own low self-worth and desperate need for your emotional provisions. The mirage is quite strong, and it's equitably constructed by your own intense longing for validation. I believe that the narcissist always comes back. Beware. This is why almost all psychological modalities suggest going no-contact, even when it's a parent.

After making so much effort and progress, the last thing you want is to be sucked back into the manipulative relationship and start from scratch. If the narcissist doesn't come back, don't take this as an offense or rejection. It is a blessing in disguise, and it means that he's making someone else's life miserable.

When I found out that the narcissist was in a relationship with someone else, my first reaction was feeling hurt and doubtful. I questioned myself and I wondered whether he was really in love with her and treating her with respect, maybe with her he was different. It didn't take too long to get my questions answered. After I decided to leave him for good, I foolishly convinced myself that I could meet him as friends. We had met a few times while he was already with her, and he kept trying to get intimate with me. Looking back, I realize how completely insane this sounds. Why the hell would I want to be friends with someone who traumatized me? Trauma bonding.

We met a few times, and I must admit that we still managed to have fun together. We laughed and had interesting conversations; it seemed like the spark was coming back again. Of course, he saw this as an opportunity to try to get me into bed with him once again. However, this time I was a different person. I had been doing the inner work, I improved the relationship with myself, and I educated myself about narcissistic personality disorder. So this time I managed to refuse him and I didn't fall for his charm. I felt repulsed, yet slightly relieved. A part of me felt bad for his new girlfriend, but at the same time, I confirmed to myself that this is who he was. And all that happened was not because of me, but because of who he is as a person. This experience gave me a sense of freedom, and I let go of any self-doubt that was tormenting me.

Reconnecting with the narcissist and feeling free from them is a great outcome for Grace. In general, I repeat, beware. Grace had done an inordinate amount of work on herself before seeing him. Remember, they will turn on all their charms and manipulations, be easy going and curious, even tender and loving, everything you ever wanted them to be. This serves two purposes: first, proving that you're still captivated by them and hence dominatable; and second, testing if you still have supply for their own desperation. I will take this a step further. If you decide to reconnect with the narcissist, check inside yourself, ask yourself directly, if there is also a need on your part to prove that you can withstand the proximity? If their wanting you back gives you a sense of power or dominance? And lastly, if it marks a measurement of your healing, like it did for Grace, which can also feel quite gratifying.

Know that the decision to be the one who no longer wants to live in suffering and in the trauma bonding culture is very disruptive if you come from that particular ecosystem. It may be disruptive to you as you heal because you will break free from your role as savior and fixer; you are hence simultaneously breaking the shackles of co-dependency, and may find yourself feeling very confused and alone without this role...at first. You will wonder what makes you lovable or valuable if you are not that. You will discover, little by little, that your joy, enthusiasm, zest for life, and laughter make you exponentially valuable, but that takes time to emotionally and psychologically substitute.

Prepare that it may also disrupt your whole original ecosystem, and you will get backlash. Your family and culture may see you as the abandoner, as the "uppity" one, maybe as even the "cold and non-compassionate" one once you place boundaries. Your successes, expansions, and determination to get better, live better, and love better may be labeled superficial and non-realistic since what is truly "real" is suffering. You may be asked to prove your suffering and show your suffering scars in order to be accepted into certain groups. I was called "Pollyanna" once because of my commitment to joy, and at the time, I felt compelled to explain that I had been sexually abused, neglected, and emotionally molested in order to justify my desire for a calm, safe, joyous adult life. The journey from trauma surviving to trauma rising is a long and arduous one. You do not have to show your medals for it. You can just reach the finish line with many of us cheering for your courage, success, and commitment to live in abundance. You get to be happy. Full stop.

Throughout my experience and educational knowledge, I have learned that narcissists have a hard time accepting the fact that you're okay without them; it hurts their ego. So, no matter what they say to try and lure you back in, remind yourself that it's not because they really love you, but because they need you for narcissistic supply. When you are vulnerable and emotionally attached to someone the moment they show some level of improvement, you might fall for their games and believe that they could actually change. As you have already witnessed in your relationship, the phase of improved behavior is only temporary, and it's only a matter of time until the narcissist takes it to another level. Each time you accept the abuser back into your life, you are sending out the message that they can get away with anything. The narcissist will never play by your rules, even though they might try to make you believe so.

Breaking the trauma bond won't happen overnight, so the sooner you stop all contact with the narcissist, the better. Once you stop seeing the narcissist, the worst is over, as you are no longer exposed to the abuse. With support and by learning how to take care of yourself, you will find yourself again and become more resilient than ever before. Becoming aware of the addictive nature of trauma bonding and the effects of intermittent reinforcement helps you understand why you feel so hooked on the narcissist. When you break the bonds that tether you to your abuser, you will open yourself up to a life free of abuse and mistreatment, and you give yourself the opportunity to develop healthy relationships and friendships that nourish you, not deplete and exploit you.

Steps to Break Free from Trauma Bonding

Step 1: Recognize that it's not love, it's trauma bonding.
Once you become aware of the trauma bond, you're less likely to fall for the narcissist's charm. Instead of telling yourself that you're staying in the relationship because of love, acknowledge that you are experiencing trauma bonding. When you change the story that you are telling yourself from a "love story" to an abusive one, you'll start seeing the relationship from a different perspective.

Step 2: Write down your thoughts and emotions.
Being in an abusive narcissistic relationship is extremely confusing and overwhelming. Writing down experiences and how they made you feel can help you become aware of patterns and manipulative lies that may not have seemed abusive in the moment. Journaling also helps you to validate your experiences and emotions denied by the narcissist.

Step 3: Observe the relationship from a different perspective.
Being emotionally involved and attached to a person makes it more difficult to see things clearly. If you had a dear friend or family member going through the same experiences you are going through, what kind of advice would you give them? Does this kind of relationship sound healthy and worth fighting for? Would it be in their best interest to stay in this kind of relationship?

Step 4: Stop all kinds of communication with the narcissist.
If you stay in contact with the narcissist, you're just making it harder for yourself to get over trauma bonding. Narcissists can be very convincing and manipulative. To gain clarity, you need to remove them from your life so you can reclaim yourself and start thinking clearly. If you have children with the narcissist, only engage in necessary conversations like when to pick the kids up, etc. Don't fall into the temptation of having conversations or trying to get them to reason things out. You're just wasting your time and energy, which will leave you feeling frustrated.

Step 5: Practice self-love and setting boundaries.
Focus on the relationship with yourself and start nourishing yourself with love and compassion. Engage in activities that bring you joy and that make you feel good about your being. Start attending to your needs and practicing setting boundaries. This will help you strengthen yourself and protect yourself from further harm and abuse.

Step 6: Surround yourself with good friends and family.
Instead of wasting your time and energy on people who belittle you, surround yourself with people who love you and truly care about you. By seeking comfort and support from people who want the best for you, you will find strength and feel less isolated. A positive environment and a good support system can do wonders to help you heal and get over a trauma bond.

Step 7: Seek professional support.

Seeking support from a licensed professional can help you a great deal to break free from trauma bonding. You can also join narcissistic abuse recovery groups, either locally or online, where you can share your experiences with other victims who can truly understand what you've been through. Feeling like you're part of a community group who share similar painful experiences helps you feel understood and less isolated. By getting the right support and working on yourself, you will get over the trauma bond and will be able to put this experience behind you.

My share in the case of breaking free from trauma bonding is twofold and is applicable to families as well. First, notice the types of conversations that you have with friends and families that work well and the ones that don't work. For example, in certain cultures, sharing your woes with the extended family works beautifully because people nod their heads, they ally around the common enemy of suffering, they have a shared experience, and quite importantly, they receive attention, care, and help, which perpetuates the familial habit of trauma bonding. There's a feeling of "we're in it together against this enemy, and we are joined in suffering." Can you see that this goes beyond a romantic relationship but actually permeates many cultures, ancestries, and human storylines?

I have clients confess to me that they are afraid of getting better for fear that I'll terminate the therapeutic relationship, as if I am not here to celebrate wholeheartedly in their victories! These are usually clients who were invisible, abandoned, or neglected because they were "fine"; better yet, they were the parentified children and were used as a supply for the needs of the suffering parent. These were children who were not rewarded for doing well but were rather abandoned or invisible. Suffering was the way to belong and to be cared for. Getting better, succeeding, excelling, or expanding made you "better than them," "Who do you think you are?"

and "You're abandoning us" by not wanting to suffer. Notice the types of conversations that work in your family or culture. Trauma bonding may be central to your ecosystem, and hence, you will seek out folks to save from their suffering or who just live in suffering, and thus the pattern will feel familiar.

- **INSIGHTFUL LESSON:** You're not in love, you're trauma bonded. When you stop romanticizing your abusive relationship you realize how toxic and damaging it really is.

Chapter 16

Grieving & Letting Go

YOU KNOW THE FEELING you have when someone really close to you passes away? That's exactly how it felt when I left the narcissist for good and started my healing journey. Realizing that what I was going through felt a lot like grieving took me by surprise. Until I had learned later on through a narcissistic abuse recovery community group that everyone experiences some form of grieving when breaking up with a narcissist.

Realizing that the person you thought was your ideal partner and knight in shining armor was actually an illusion hits you hard. It takes time for your mind to process the fact that the person you thought you loved was nothing but a fictional character projected by the narcissist to hook you and trap you into a manipulative relationship. Even though this person doesn't really exist, for you, all that you experienced during the love bombing phase was very real. You feel hurt, tricked, and you have to somehow find a way to accept that you were living a lie.

This is what makes breaking free from a narcissist so mentally and emotionally exhausting—it creates a deep internal conflict known as cognitive dissonance. Your mind struggles to reconcile two opposing truths: the loving, caring person you thought they were, and the manipulative, hurtful reality you've come to see. One part of you clings to the beautiful memories, the charm, and the promises, while the other part slowly begins to accept the painful truth that none of it was real. This contradiction leaves you feeling emotionally paralyzed, confused, and stuck in a cycle of denial and hope, unable to fully let go.

Understanding that the love bombing phase was not genuine, but it was actually a trap, leaves you feeling terrified, and you lose the ability to trust others and yourself. This is something that haunted me for months. If what I perceived to be true was actually fake, then how was I going to be able to tell what was actually real from that point onwards? Coming to terms with the fact that this ideal character he created at the beginning of our relationship was an illusion was not easy. But I wanted to be free of suffering, and I understood that I had no other option but to find a way to let go of this imaginary person.

I looked back at myself and how I had behaved in the relationship, and I felt foolish and embarrassed, seeing the lengths I had gone through to try to make things work. I now realize that much of my suffering came from resisting what was, instead of accepting it. I was trying to force something that was never meant to be, clinging to an illusion, and exhausting myself in the process. In hindsight, I now see how this struggle reflects an ancient Taoist principle—one that, had I embraced earlier, could have saved me from immense suffering. This practice is called Wu Wei, the art of effortless action.

Wu Wei teaches us that true peace comes not from control or force, but from aligning with and flowing with the natural course of life, rather than resisting it. Reflecting on my past, I see how life was constantly nudging me to let go, yet I refused to listen. There were countless red flags, but the more I ignored them, the louder they became. It reached a point where I even experienced physical accidents, like the one I had in Budapest, all because I was desperately holding onto something that was actively breaking me.

This practical philosophy is about surrendering to life's natural flow and trusting that what resists us is often not meant for us. It does not mean passivity or giving up; it means recognizing when to stop fighting against the current and allowing things to unfold as they are meant to. Learning to trust the flow of life, rather than trying to control it, became one of the most profound lessons of my healing journey.

Throughout my grieving phase, I learned how to accept the fact that I could never have a true, loving, and intimate relationship with a narcissist.

Likening this stage to a death is exact. It is a death of the fantasy, a death of who you thought you were, a death of who you thought you were together, and a death to who you have been in relationships—all of your relationships thus far. It is an identity death. Who are you now, without trauma bonding, without volatility, without living close to the edge? How are you to do love, sex, intimacy, and relationships now?

This stage is a chrysalis. What most people don't know about a chrysalis is that the caterpillar actually turns into goo inside the chrysalis; it does not shed, it becomes amorphous. It literally goes from being goo to form into something new entirely, a butterfly. This period of grief—and I love that Grace speaks to it so we can normalize it and include it as an actual step on the healing journey—is a time to disintegrate the old self. It is a time to press rewind on your childhood videotapes, study your attachment style, and comprehend your relational culture and language. It is a time for a sacred pause.

I love grief. Grief is active. Grief is what mothers do at the Wailing Wall in Jerusalem, as they rock back and forth in mourning. Humans wail, howl, curl up into the fetal position, and kneel as they grieve. Grief has the possibility of high alchemy if it's used to sear the wound into a healed scar. Grace also speaks to the fact that we can hold multiple feelings at the same time: we can feel hatred and repulsion for the abuser, and we can feel sadness, grief, and even longing for what could have been. Herein lies the importance of honoring the feelings that arise; allowing them to come up non-judgmentally and mindfully serves as the transmutation that gives way to the transformation (OTTE: observe, transmute, transform, evolve). Here, here, grieving chrysalis.

The process of grieving and letting go took me a significant amount of time. Through meditation, psychotherapy, and other somatic healing techniques, I managed to find a way to allow myself to feel whatever I needed to feel so I could be free from these painful emotions and move on to the next chapter of my life. Allowing myself to feel these emotions was indeed painful, but I made a pact with myself that I would never allow someone to hurt me like that ever again. Not getting any kind of closure from the narcissist made it more difficult to let go and move on. I had found myself trying to get him to understand the pain he had caused me. No matter how hard I tried to make him realize, he couldn't be bothered, and he refused to acknowledge what he did or give me any kind of closure whatsoever. I realized that the only person who could give me closure was myself.

In my tenure as a psychotherapist, I find the process of getting closure on your own, without a bilateral process, one of the most arduous, painful, and tumultuous psychological undertakings to endure. It can also be a high spiritual portal if one can complete the closure within a loving, witnessing environment. It is more common that not to not have closure and some examples of this are a parent that stays alcoholic, an ex who happily remarries, a sexual abuser that is alive and systemically protected, or died and you are left without the right to confront them, and a life in a subjugating culture where the abuser is supported and not confronted for fear of them.

Slavery, Jim Crow, Jeffrey Epstein, cults, are all examples of narcissistic systems, abuses, and non-closures. This high-level, deep-diving, self-facing internal spelunking is not for the faint of heart, but as Grace attests, support groups, therapists, therapy groups, coaches, books, journals, and lots of kneeling and grieving will do the work. When working with clients who are doing closures on their own, the "why" stage lasts a while. Why did this happen? Why were they like this? Why did they treat me this way? Why didn't they love me? Why were they so cruel? Why wasn't I protected? Why didn't anyone do anything? Why? The why stage is necessary, lengthy, and requires much grief.

Have heart: on the other side of the long "why tunnel" awaits the yellow ribbon of closure, and it sounds something like "Why no longer matters; that's them and this is me. I love myself and I vow to love myself even more. I vow not to let this happen again. It is me who closes this chapter. It is me who writes my story." Closure. Grace found it, and this book is a testimony. This is what we mean spiritually as transcendence, a very high place indeed.

I accepted the fact that due to his personality disorder, he was not able to empathize with me or own up to his mistakes.

I find Grace's approach of not taking it personally by acknowledging that he has a personality disorder helpful, particularly for Empaths. The Empath tends to see the other's point of view with great ease and wisdom, is sensitive and feels the other's pain and wound, even as they are themselves being wounded. This will often make it difficult to leave or have closure because the instinct to save, heal, or fix can be quite compulsive.

Understanding that this is a personality disorder objectifies the behavior, removes it from being personalized, and grants permission to separate oneself from the need to save or fix. A parallel spiritual process that "depersonalizes" and aids in decreasing the co-dependency to the Narcissist's wounded past, is to fully realize that we are all on our life journey and our individual journey has unique teachings for each of us.

Yes, we are here together and some spiritual philosophies hold that we chose to come into this lifetime together to either close karmic loops or learn the lessons we need to learn in order to evolve, and yet, we are here on our individual journey and who we journey with at each stretch may and will change.

I find it very helpful for my Empath heart to understand that each of us are floating between concentric circles and we will shift and move between them according to our learnings. None is better, superior, above, below, or inferior; we are all hitting spots on the journey where we either move to our next teaching or not. What determines our evolution is our faith in more love, more growth, more peace as well as the tools, guides, and fellow journeyers to swim through life's emotional and psychological tsunamis. If you're reading this, you, Grace, and I are meeting at a mutual concentric circle and are journeying together through this very moment in time. You are not abandoning the narcissist; you are allowing them to have their own journey.

He continued to project everything on me and blamed me for everything that went wrong in our relationship. Knowing that he was not able to accept his own imperfections and obnoxious personality traits gave me the closure that I needed. I stopped taking this personally and blaming myself for not being the perfect person he wanted me to be. Working on the relationship with myself was the best decision I could have made as it allowed me to free myself from his tormenting words.

Steps to Letting Go & Moving Forward

Step 1: Let go of internalizing the narcissist's behavior.
Remind yourself that their actions were never about you not being good enough, pretty enough, strong enough, rich enough, or anything else. How people behave is a reflection of them, not of you. Their inability to love, respect, or value you has nothing to do with your worth as an individual. You were simply caught in the crossfire of their own inner wounds and dysfunction. Free yourself from the false belief that their mistreatment was a result of your inadequacy.

Step 2: Let go of the need to be "good enough."
Stop trying to prove yourself to the narcissist in hopes of gaining their approval or validation. The harsh truth is that you could never be "good enough" for someone who is wired to shift blame, avoid accountability, and project their insecurities onto others. Recognize that your worth is not dependent on their distorted perception of you. True healing begins when you decide that you are enough without their validation.

Step 3: Let go of what other people think.
Worrying about the judgment of family, mutual friends, their family, your children, colleagues, or anyone else can make leaving and healing more complicated. But the truth is, their opinions do not define you. Your happiness, peace, and well-being carry far more value than the approval of others. Letting go of the need to be understood or accepted by everyone will free you to make choices that align with your highest good.

Step 4: Let go of the version of yourself you created to please others.
When we struggle with people-pleasing tendencies and seek love and validation externally, we become inauthentic and lose sight of who we truly are. We compromise our needs, boundaries, and values just to fit into an image that makes others comfortable. It's time to return to yourself.

Embrace the journey of self-discovery, unlearning the conditioning that shaped you, and peeling back the layers to reveal your authentic essence.

Step 5: Let go of false hope.
Holding onto the hope that the narcissist will change, heal, give you closure, or validate your experience only keeps you stuck in their cycle. They will not wake up one day and suddenly treat you with the love and respect you deserve. Instead of hoping for their transformation, shift your hope toward your own future. The one where you heal, thrive, and experience the love, peace, and joy you were always meant to have.

Step 6: Let go of anger and resentment, find forgiveness.
Feeling anger after betrayal is natural; it signals that your boundaries were violated. Acknowledge this anger, but don't let it consume you. Holding onto resentment does not punish them; it only poisons you. It blocks your inner peace, weighs down your spirit, and even affects your physical health.

Forgiveness doesn't mean reconciliation or excusing their actions. It means choosing to no longer carry the burden of their actions in your heart. It means understanding their dysfunction without letting it define you. By releasing anger, you free yourself from their chaos while they remain trapped in their own destructive patterns.

Forgiveness is about making peace with the past, rather than staying trapped in regret. It's about processing your experiences, learning from them, and transmuting that pain into growth and transformation. Release your anger and resentment for your own sake, so you don't carry the weight of their actions into the next chapter of your life.

Embrace Somatic Practices for Release

Even after leaving the relationship and starting my healing journey, I didn't realize that shame and anger were still trapped in my body. My journey took an unexpected turn when I began experiencing unexplained muscle twitches—first in my eyelids, then spreading to various parts of my body. Despite thorough medical checks, the cause remained a mystery, leading to a diagnosis of stress-related symptoms.

The breakthrough came unexpectedly at a cacao ceremony and ecstatic dance. Skeptical yet curious, I had no particular expectations. However, upon consuming the cacao, a profound realization hit me: I was carrying immense pain internally. This insight unleashed a flood of painful memories, and as I danced, I wept, allowing myself to feel and process my emotions fully. Remarkably, the mysterious twitches disappeared after this profound emotional release.

This experience led me to explore somatic release and therapy. According to the Harvard Health Blog ("What is somatic therapy?", n.d.), somatic therapy offers a holistic approach to addressing trauma. This discovery was pivotal in my healing, addressing not just the mind and spirit but the body as well. I strongly encourage exploring somatic practices as they might just be the key to unlocking and releasing deep-seated pain.

Journal Prompts

Describe an experience, a memory, or a feeling that you would like to let go of today.

What thoughts, emotions, and energy would you like to invite into your life in place of what you're releasing?

Write down three positive affirmations that resonate with you and help cultivate a sense of peace, confidence, and self-worth. Keep a journal beside your bed and repeat these affirmations every morning and before you sleep, with intention!

What valuable lesson has this experience taught you about yourself, your needs, or your boundaries?

Write a Letter

Place one hand on your heart and the other on your stomach. Take three deep, mindful breaths, allowing yourself to be fully present with your emotions, with loving kindness and compassion.

When you're ready, write a letter to the narcissist, expressing everything you have ever wanted to say. Let your emotions flow freely onto the page—anger, grief, disappointment, or even moments of clarity. Say the things you never got the chance to, without holding back.

This letter is not meant to be sent. It is for you, not for them. Writing is a tool for release—to free yourself from the weight of unspoken words and transform the emotional energy into something tangible, allowing you to process and transcend it.

Dolores Cannon, a metaphysical therapist, seeker, and researcher, describes a beautiful psychospiritual approach to breaking a karmic loop, closing a relationship, cutting an ancestral bond, or ending what she calls a "soul contract." One way to break free from karmic lessons is by learning the lesson in each experience of suffering, in other words, by deepening our self-understanding and by upleveling out of the suffering through self-growth and self-love.

This is what we call consciousness. When we find ourselves in a repetitive cycle of a particular experience or with a particular person, we are caught in a karmic loop where we are not able to see the lesson directly, and so we cannot uplevel into consciousness from it. Like Grace's letter, Dolores Cannon suggests spiritually breaking your soul contract with that person or lesson, by either writing it down and tearing it up, or visualizing actually tearing it up.

It goes something like this: bring the person or experience into your mind; feel the repetitive feelings you have from them; visualize the contract between you wherein was written the lesson you were meant to learn together; feel yourself tearing the contract up in many pieces; speak your truth to this person and say, "We tried, we really tried and it didn't work. Let's tear up this contract. Now we can stop." Do this with honesty and conviction. Then say, "I forgive you. I release you. I let you go. I forgive myself. I release me. I let me go. You go away with love, and I go my way. We don't have to be connected anymore." Feel the release of allowing yourself this freedom and forgive your part in this soul contract.

I encourage using this with a relationship that may feel like a contract with suffering or poverty. Tear up that contract and say, "I release you and let you go." By believing in this process, you are breaking the energetic ties that bound you to this person; I would even expand it to the role you decided to play with yourself. This exercise, when done with belief and conviction, is a path to higher consciousness.

Chapter 17

Discovering Who You Really Are

THE RELATIONSHIP WITH THE narcissist consumed all my time and energy. From the moment I opened my eyes until I went to sleep, I was entirely focused on the relationship. I devoted myself to making everything perfect and tiptoed around him to avoid triggering him. Suddenly, I had no one to nurture, no one to take care of, and nothing to distract me from turning inward and facing myself.

It was terrifying yet simultaneously relieving. I realized that I had spent the past decade focusing on saving others instead of getting to know who I was, what I had to offer, why I came into this world, and what wounds I needed to heal. I felt isolated and like I didn't belong anywhere or with anyone. In the first few months of being alone, I was carried away by whatever came my way. I went to places which made me feel like an outsider. I hung out with people who supported me, but I was still struggling to find my place, a true connection, and a sense of belonging.

Months passed by, and I was still feeling empty and lost. To distract myself from my own demons, I started working endless hours, and at some point, I almost lived in the office of the company I was working for. I was immersed in the world of private aviation. An industry of luxury, materialism, and glamour. Focusing on work helped me escape the tormenting thoughts and the void within me. I was thriving in my career, and this helped me boost my self-confidence as I started believing in myself and embracing my skills and capabilities.

Finding meaning, purpose, and self-confidence in work was Grace's way of sublimating, a psychological behavior I value and appreciate. It's a way of using negative energy—feeling lost and isolated—and channeling it into something that will ultimately feel constructive and self-edifying. Work served as an anchor while she mulled these identity questions around.

However, even though I was succeeding professionally, I remember sitting alone in my living room and wondering why I still felt so empty inside. No matter how much I achieved, I couldn't shake the feeling that I didn't belong anywhere—a feeling that had been tormenting me since childhood.

Looking back, the answer seems obvious. How can you understand where you belong if you don't even know who you really are? How do you expect to belong if you hang out at the wrong places with the wrong people? Back then, it didn't seem so obvious. I was too busy trying to run away from the wounds that resided within me. Work was all that mattered to me at that point, but life found a way to put me in my place and forced me to go within myself. This time, I had nowhere to escape.

Using an external process or substance in order to escape our internal world is a coping mechanism, a defense, at worst, an addiction, and always, a common human response to difficult feelings. It begins as an adaptive response to something that feels unbearable. Defenses are there to protect us children, but they become overbearing life usurpers with time. Have compassion for their origin, and courage for their dismantling.

I was thriving in my career when the world experienced a pandemic outbreak. Everyone's world turned upside down as COVID-19 spread across the four corners of the world faster than wildfire. Back then, I remember thinking that this was the last thing I needed. Considering that I was trying to heal my emotional trauma, find myself, and build a solid foundation for my life, I was already carrying a heavy emotional burden. Dealing with the fear and stress of a global pandemic only added to my anxiety and depression, making everything feel even more overwhelming. Little did I know that from this point onwards, my whole life would change forever.

Quite soon after the pandemic broke out, I lost my job, and it felt like my whole world had been shattered once again. It was the only thing keeping me sane at the time, taking away all my time, energy, and attention so I didn't have to focus on myself. But life decided to shake up my world once again and redirected me towards my highest path. However, at the time, I wasn't aware of this, and I couldn't make sense out of my suffering. When you're in a dark place, you struggle to see the light, and it's easy to fall into the trap of self-victimization. I felt like I had hit rock bottom. I was working hard to try and build up my self-confidence and become self-reliant, and somehow everything was taken away from me. I felt so angry at life and was drowning in self-pity. I would lie down on the floor in my apartment and just cry for hours, feeling completely helpless and broken.

Around the same time I lost my job, I had to spend 14 days in mandatory self-quarantine after being repatriated to Europe from the United States, where I had been working. Throughout these 14 days of self-quarantine, I had quite a lot of time on my hands to reflect on myself and retreat inward. So, I decided to find solace in meditation and continued my practice as my healer had taught me.

This experience of "going in" during the pandemic—physically and emotionally—wreaked havoc, shook emotional fault lines, stirred up ancestral ghosts, and catapulted thousands of people all over the planet into a spiritual awakening that is unprecedented. The good, the bad, the ugly, and the divine emerged and gave rise to a world where discussion around trauma, healing, and spirituality are center stage and constant. This post-pandemic era is rife with wounding and separatism, as well as replete with ascension, transcendence, and possibility.

It harkens us to Dickens' words, "it was the best of times and it was the worst of times." We are in the tale of two worlds, and I find that personal evolution, like Grace's, is paving the road to collective evolution for this emerging era.

In the first week of quarantine, I was going through my staff cleaning and organizing the house to kill some time. I found a few books that had accumulated dust on them as I hadn't looked at them for years. One of these books stood out to me. I had no idea what it was about as I didn't really understand the title. I read the summary at the back of the book, and I didn't really get what it was about either. I couldn't explain why or how, but I felt called to read it. I had received this book from my ex-narcissist's mum about two years before, but I had never intended to read it. I didn't know that my higher self was guiding me to read this book, and I didn't realize how divinely timed this moment was until I started reading it.

What a beautiful example of Grace's inner being or her intuition leading her to what was best for her. We see this inner voice show up in many ways during her narcissistic travesty, and it's beautiful to see it show up again. We are not alone on this life journey, even when it seems like we are. Noticing, tracking, and highlighting these moments assist in the construction of a spiritually abundant escrow and lighthouse for the rest of the journey.

The first time I started reading this book, I was in bed before going to sleep. I had never heard of the author Eckhart Tolle, so I had no idea what to expect. The book had a strange title: *A New Earth.* Before I started reading the first page, I remember saying to myself how strange the title sounded, and wondering what the author meant by it. So, I decided to dive into this book and see what it's all about. By the time I had read the first few pages, the strangest thing happened to me. I felt like an explosion of energy starting from my tailbone, going up my spine, and the feeling was so powerful that it gave me goosebumps. I was startled in bed, I paused, put the book down, and wondered what was happening to me. I took a look at my body and I saw my skin still covered with goosebumps.

Grace's response to Eckhart Tolle's book is what I call a full-chakra light up! It is a holistic response—mind, body, heart, and spirit—to a multidimensional awareness. It feels like spiritual eroticism, and what I mean by that is the experience of full communion between the material and spiritual world, a wondrous love making, if you will, where the invisible and the visible become one. So many prophets have written about this divine love-making, like Theresa D'Avila, a 15th-century nun who described herself as being in ecstatic love for God, "It is a caressing of love so sweet which now takes place between the soul and God." (from her autobiography).

Grace had a soulful and mystical sensation that rippled through her body. This moment can also be described as a moment where she recognized her full self in the work or eyes of another.

I continued reading, and I was having these powerful moments of realization about life and suffering, about our human experience, and I suddenly had a deeper understanding of life in general. It felt like an expansion of awareness, and the energetic movement from my tailbone going up my spine continued for several minutes, giving me goosebumps. For the first time in my life, I realized that I was sensing my own spirit moving through me, the Life force energy that was keeping my body up and running. Later on, I discovered that this is called Kundalini energy, a powerful spiritual force lying dormant at the base of the spine. When awakened, it rises through the body, leading to expanded awareness and transformation.

Prior to this experience, I was a strong-headed atheist, firmly rejecting anything spiritual. But feeling my own spirit moving within me was undeniable. For the first time ever, I realized that I was more than just my physical body. And so, the veil was lifted.

This description of her organic, spiritual awakening is sublime. Yes, the veil has lifted all over the planet. There is a spiritual renaissance that is calling us to a higher life experience and the birthing of a new world. Hark, the herald angels sing.

The following morning, I woke up feeling strangely energized, despite having barely slept. As I got out of bed and opened the curtains, I noticed something shocking. My double-glazed window was broken from the inside. The outer glass was intact, but the inner layer had completely shattered. I had no explanation for it.

A few days later, as I continued diving deeper into my meditation and reflections, another bizarre event occurred. While carefully washing dishes, I placed a glass lid on the counter, and right before my eyes, it cracked and shattered into pieces. These experiences blew my mind. I felt confused and scared, and I had this inner knowing that something beyond my understanding was unfolding before me.

I felt a strong curiosity and a compelling need to understand what was happening to me. So, I began researching Eckhart Tolle, his books, and his teachings. That's when I found myself immersed in a whole new world—a new reality. I had never finished reading a book so quickly, and from that point onward, I felt like I was reborn into a new person.

As I continued learning about these mystical encounters, I discovered that many people who read the book went through the same experience, which they called a *"spiritual awakening."* This expansion of consciousness and enhanced awareness allowed me to understand the purpose behind my suffering. All of a sudden, everything made sense to me. All the suffering that I had been through and the continuous turbulence in my life served a purpose. I realized that I was exactly where I needed to be and that everything was divinely timed.

Indeed, the Christian sequence of Jesus' suffering on Friday, followed by a silent Saturday of profound reckoning, into the Easter Sunday of resurrection, is what grace is describing here. Her suffering led her to her internal, reflective self, which is now being resurrected into her emerging, empowered self, with the help of the Holy Spirit. I use a Christian reference here only as one example of many. Buddha followed a similar sequence of experiencing multiple paths in life, including one where he suffered, and through it, he surfaced on the other side into Enlightenment. The description of the chrysalis also works well.

There are many metaphors for this human experience of passionate communion with the divine. The juxtaposition of suffering prior to resurrecting is not lost here, where the wound is the portal to the gift. This is my personal definition of heaven on earth, a continuous alchemical process of curating our moment-by-moment experience by understanding suffering as possibility. Heaven on earth is reaching for the celestial while adoring the earthly.

Going through this spiritual awakening transformed me, and my whole life changed forever. Later on, I learned that many people who go through narcissistic abuse may also have this experience. Narcissistic abuse forces you to go within yourself and seek the truth to learn who you really are through Gnosis—a deep, experiential knowledge of spiritual truth that goes beyond intellectual understanding. It is the kind of wisdom that comes from direct inner realization, rather than external teachings alone.

Now, of course, this does not justify or glorify narcissists. Causing someone pain and emotional turmoil is unacceptable and should not be tolerated in any circumstances. But seeing that these kinds of experiences serve a bigger purpose helps you grow and evolve as a person. It helps you to stop victimizing yourself, learn, and move forward. Whether you experience a spiritual awakening or not doesn't really matter. What matters is that you take a step back and reflect on what kind of lessons you need to learn from this experience.

Becoming in touch with your true essence unleashes an unstoppable power that you never knew you had within you. Regardless of what religion or belief system you identify with, recognizing the infinite intelligence that sustains you opens both your mind and heart to a new reality. This inner force is far more powerful than flesh and bones. It holds the key to resilience, transformation, and renewal.

Like the phoenix, you have the power to rise from the ashes of your past, reborn into a stronger and more authentic version of yourself. But true transformation requires letting go of what no longer serves you. To heal and allow your true self to emerge, you must distance yourself from the abuser.

I've come to understand that everything happens for a reason, even if, in the moment, we struggle to find meaning in our suffering. In the ancient alchemical process, transformation begins with the "Negredo" stage, symbolizing the darkness, dissolution, and breaking down of the old self. Though painful, this stage is necessary to clear away illusions, much like how fire refines gold. Through self-awareness, we gain the wisdom to alchemize our pain into growth and, eventually, see the bigger picture.

Journaling for Self-Reflection

Journaling has been a deeply insightful practice for me, allowing me to look back and see how much I've grown over time. It's like having a written record of my transformation, witnessing how my thoughts, emotions, and actions have evolved.

I encourage you to start journaling, even if you don't consider yourself a "writer." Write as if you were speaking to your closest, most trusted friend. Let your journal be a safe space where you can express your feelings without fear of judgment.

Journaling is especially powerful when you're feeling overwhelmed. Putting your thoughts into words helps you organize your emotions, gain clarity, and release heavy energy. And if you commit to writing just once a month, by the end of the year, you'll have written 12 chapters of your life—a tangible reflection of your journey.

Journal Prompts

Use these prompts to deepen your self-awareness and uncover what truly resonates with you.

What comes naturally to me? (e.g., painting, singing, cooking, dancing, connecting with others, problem-solving)

What skills do I want to learn and develop?

What kind of places do I enjoy spending time in? Why?

What are my interests, and is there anything I would like to contribute to?

What would I regret not doing before my time here is over?

How do I envision my life a year from now? What changes would I like to see?

What are my long-term goals, and what impact do I want to create in my life?

How can I break these long-term goals into smaller, achievable steps?

How do I intend to show up for myself in order to bring this vision to life and manifest it?

How can I take better care of myself and meet my own needs, rather than waiting for others to fulfill them?

Write a Letter to Yourself

Put one hand on your heart and one hand on your stomach. Take 3 deep, mindful breaths. Write a letter to yourself and write down whatever needs to come out. Give yourself permission to express yourself freely with yourself. You are safe in this space.

Chapter 18

Falling In Love With Yourself

ACCORDING TO A NEWS article on News18 (n.d.), a survey has identified a self-love crisis that is prevalent worldwide ("Survey Identifies Self-Love Crisis Around the World"). It's ironic how something so vital to our happiness and fulfillment in life can be so difficult to cultivate and embody. The fact that I ended up in abusive relationships strongly reflected that I was already struggling with self-love. And being in a relationship with a narcissist didn't make it any easier for me. Learning how to fall in love with myself required work, effort, and commitment. But when you think about it, any kind of relationship requires work, effort, and commitment. So why not dedicate some time to improving the relationship with yourself?

The world being in a self-love crisis makes perfect sense and is quite precise. The collective has not been taught to self-love and much less to feel securely attached. In fact, humanity's recorded history—and still today—is full of the story of narcissistic systems subjugating humans. Dominance through hierarchical fear has been the running human philosophy since Cain and

Abel. I posit that self-hate is at the root of all personal dysfunctions, abuse, mental illness, and physical diseases. The world is a collective representation of the individual's journey.

In the previous chapter, I made a parallel with Grace's awakening and the planet's awakening post-pandemic. The collective is learning about itself, facing its trauma, searching for healing, insisting on self-love, and yearning to start anew. As I clearly state on my website's homepage and my book The Empath Leader, *the planet is needing some secure parenting right about now. There is an antidote to the narcissistic model, and it starts with you.*

Throughout my healing journey, I decided that I would start dating myself, and I started getting curious about who I really was as a human being. It was scary, especially at the beginning, but isn't every relationship a bit scary in the beginning? When you start dating someone, you're not sure whether you will like the person or not. So I thought to myself that whatever I found that I didn't like about myself, I could work on and improve to become a better version of myself. Now, of course, self-acceptance is key to cultivating self-love. Accepting yourself as you are means that you love yourself despite your imperfections and whatever you might not like about yourself. But self-acceptance doesn't mean that you're not allowed to improve yourself as a person.

On the other hand, rejecting the parts of yourself that you don't like will only fuel negative thoughts and emotions toward yourself. This internal conflict creates deep wounds in your psyche, a concept that psychiatrist Carl Jung referred to as The Shadow—the hidden, repressed aspects of ourselves that we struggle to accept. When we reject these parts, we create a split within our being, further fragmenting ourselves rather than working toward integration and wholeness. True healing comes from acknowledging, understanding, and embracing all parts of who we are, even the ones we've been conditioned to hide.

Boy, oh boy, was this journey difficult for me. It took a tremendous amount of effort to cleanse myself of the belittling comments the narcissist had implanted in my mind. Even more challenging was digging deeper into the deep-rooted emotional wounds that existed long before I met him—the very wounds that shaped me into the perfect match for a narcissist.

But I made it a point to prove to myself that he was not right about me. I refused to let his distorted version of me define who I was. So, I made myself the most important project of my life. I started challenging myself, stepping outside of my comfort zone, and doing things that scared me. It was uncomfortable, but it was necessary. I understood that I needed to face my demons and my biggest fears to overcome them and become a stronger person. I wanted to break free from feeling codependent on others, and I craved to feel free and self-reliant. With every challenge that I overcame, I felt empowered, free, and more resilient. During this process, I learned a lot about myself. It became clear to me that I was holding on to the narcissist because I was scared that he was the best I could do. The narcissist was reflecting back to me everything that I deeply believed about myself. My lack of self-worth and fear of abandonment made me feel helpless, and I was willing to do anything to avoid being abandoned.

It's important to highlight this cognitive distortion: this person may be the best I can do. It is such a common belief, and it keeps us from leaving abusive situations! Highlight this thought and do the work to delete it. Grace is showing the clear example that the best you can do is precisely in your very hands. The best you can do is YOU. Loving you first and foremost is the best you can do, and what's better, it does not rely on another person. Ideally, we would have been born into homes where we felt adored and securely attached, but that is not the case for most humans, simply because the generations preceding this one did not know how to. Humans are evolving, and they are evolving into self-love and are learning the tools and processes for it. Self-exploration, self-healing, self-love, and secure attachment are the name of the game, and again, it starts with you.

When I started dating myself, I learned how to enjoy being with my own company, which helped me overcome the fear of abandonment. I realized that I knew how to make myself happy: I discovered what I enjoyed doing and what I was truly passionate about. I finally had the time to explore myself and allow my authentic self to emerge. The more I learned about myself, the more I started enjoying my own company to the point where I started rejecting invites to social events. I preferred to hang out with myself rather than going to places with friends just for the sake of not being alone, and I learned how to set boundaries and say no when I really wanted to say no. Falling in love with myself was an eye-opening experience as I realized that the thing that I was fearing and avoiding the most was exactly what I needed to do to be free. So you might be thinking, what does it mean to start dating yourself?

Knowing how to be alone is a skill. I don't mean loneliness that comes from abandonment and neglect. I mean learning how to creatively, lovingly, and mindfully be alone. Grace is describing it beautifully here. The art of being alone and of loving one's own company sets the groundwork for not choosing a lesser life for the fear of being alone. Loving oneself may feel ambitious and seem like a lofty ideal, but it is the most worthy and noble of endeavors.

I find that loving oneself is easier when we first declutter what makes us hate ourselves, as depicted in Grace's journey. When we do the clean-up work and carefully deconstruct the layers that buried the love with OTTE (observation, transmutation, transformation, evolution), the path to self-love becomes clearer. Grace has shown us that this endeavor requires quite a bit of personal ferocity, but I claim that it is the highest human endeavor.

Acts of Service to Yourself: Learning to Date Yourself

We tend to associate acts of service with doing things for others. We show love through thoughtful gestures, helping, and making them feel special. But what if you started showing up for yourself in the same way?

Acts of service to yourself are intentional actions that nurture, support, and prioritize your well-being. There are ways to express love, care, and appreciation for yourself, just as you would for a partner or a loved one.

Many of us wait for someone else to take us on a romantic dinner, surprise us with a trip, or cook a nourishing meal. But why should we depend on others for experiences that we are perfectly capable of creating for ourselves? The more you show up for yourself, the more you reinforce your self-worth, self-love, and confidence.

So, instead of waiting for someone to make you feel special, here are some meaningful ways to start dating yourself and show up as your own best partner.

Take Yourself Out on Coffee or Brunch Dates

Plan a date with yourself just like you would with someone you care about. Get dressed, put on something that makes you feel good, and make an event out of it. It's not just about the coffee or meal, it's about showing up for yourself with intention and presence.

Once you're there, avoid mindlessly scrolling through social media or checking emails. Treat it like a real date, so be present with yourself. Bring a book, write in your journal, or observe your surroundings. Take in the taste of your food, the warmth of the coffee, the aroma in the air, and the ambiance around you.

If sitting alone at a café feels uncomfortable at first, remind yourself that it's only your inner critic talking. People are too caught up in their own lives to judge you. And if anything, being comfortable in your own company is a sign of self-confidence and self-love.

Cook Nourishing Meals for Yourself

Many people believe that cooking a nice meal is only worth the effort if it's for someone else. But this belief sends a subtle message to yourself: "I am not worth the time and effort."

Think about how much love and energy you would put into preparing a meal for someone you care about. Now, imagine putting that same care and intention into cooking for yourself.

Choose a meal you genuinely enjoy, plate it beautifully, and set the table. Turn it into a self-care ritual rather than a chore. The way you treat yourself in small, everyday actions shapes how you see yourself. Show yourself that you are worthy of nourishment, effort, and care.

Travel Solo: Discover Yourself Through Adventure

Solo travel might seem intimidating, but it is one of the most powerful ways to connect with yourself. When you travel alone, you push beyond your comfort zone, meet new people, and learn how to rely on yourself in ways you never imagined.

When you're traveling alone, you learn what excites you, what scares you, and what truly brings you joy. You make decisions without needing to compromise, you choose where to go, what to eat, and how to spend your time.

If traveling abroad alone feels overwhelming, start small. Take a weekend trip to a nearby city or go on a solo day trip. The confidence and independence you gain from these experiences will reflect in all areas of your life.

Try New Activities & Learn Something New

Exploring new activities is a great way to get to know yourself on a deeper level. What excites you? What challenges you? What makes you feel alive?

Trying new things not only keeps life exciting but also boosts your self-esteem. It's a reminder that you are constantly growing, evolving, and capable of expanding your comfort zone.

Here are some ideas to start with:

- **Creative activities:** Painting, writing, pottery, playing an instrument.
- **Physical activities:** Dance classes, yoga, rock climbing, hiking.
- **Intellectual growth:** Taking an online course, learning a new language.
- **Pure fun experiences:** Going to an amusement park, trying karaoke, or doing something spontaneous just for the joy of it.

The goal is to explore, experiment, and enjoy yourself. You are your own best company, and the more you invest in yourself, the more fulfilled and complete you will feel.

Plan Your First Date with Yourself

Now that you have ideas for acts of service to yourself, it's time to take action! Fill in the table below and commit to your first self-date.

When will you take yourself on a date?
Date: _______________

Where will you go?
Location: _______________

What will you do?
Activity: _______________

Remember: Treat this as an important commitment to yourself. Whether you take yourself out for coffee, cook a nourishing meal, or book a solo getaway, do it with love and intention.

The most important relationship you will ever have is the one with yourself. Show up for you.

Accepting Who You Are

When you start dating someone, it's only a matter of time until you discover aspects of the person that you don't like. This doesn't hold us back from loving the other person. So why should it be any different for you?

Throughout my healing journey, I realized how exhausted I felt from trying to be perfect and always trying to avoid mistakes because of the narcissist. As our relationship evolved, he consistently tried to find new ways to make me feel ashamed of who I am. Even a simple fact like asking me about my favorite smell or favorite food. He used to shame me for not being special enough or unique in my tastes. Back then, his words used to destroy me because I valued his opinion, and I didn't value myself. Looking back, I realize how ridiculous and pointless it all was.

To free myself from these memories and the heavy emotions they inflicted, I learned how to allow myself to like whatever I truly liked, and I gave permission to myself to be who I really am. I started telling myself that it's okay not to be perfect, it's okay to make mistakes as long as you learn from them. This sense of acceptance allowed me to start viewing mistakes as learning opportunities to become better. It empowered me to try new things as I wasn't scared of failure and being rejected. I realized that I was taking life too seriously, and I became even more curious about my capabilities and my potential.

In my Empath Leader Training, I do an exercise where the participants have to study, speak about, and share their areas of genius as well as their areas of imperfection. I find Grace's acceptance work invaluable, and I would add that this work includes accepting her areas—your areas—of giftedness, of genius, of high IQ, and high EQ. It is incredibly hard to accept where we are imperfect, what Jung calls this shadow work: the process of befriending our neglected, unlikeable sides, that tend to stalk and ambush us, especially in relationships. It is equally hard, and possibly even harder, to fully befriend our magnificent sides, especially for the Empath, who may hide or become smaller in order not to intimidate the narcissist or to avoid competitive confrontation.

The work of doing both creates a profound balance that expresses itself as courageousness, just as Grace describes. It allows for boldness and risk-taking to know that we have areas of magnificence and areas where we can be imperfect. We are thus more securely attached to ourselves and are free to explore, even when we make mistakes.

This shift in my perception opened the door to new opportunities and brought about powerful changes in my life. The more I accepted myself and allowed my authentic self to emerge, the more I started meeting people who resonated with who I really am. When I started accepting myself, others seemed to be more accepting of me. Having acceptance of who I am helped me to stop wanting to impress others and pretending to be someone else. I wasn't ashamed of who I am anymore. Once you return to who you really are, you unleash the power of authenticity, which can help you create a joyful and harmonious life aligned with your true values.

What positive qualities do you embrace about yourself?

What imperfections are you ready to accept about yourself?

What emotions, thoughts, or opinions have you been hiding from others to protect yourself from being rejected?

Be Compassionate with Yourself

Narcissists are mean and demeaning, and after being exposed to their belittling comments, it's easy to end up speaking to yourself the same way. You might find yourself saying how stupid you are for falling for them. Or perhaps you start telling yourself that you're the one to blame for everything. Instead of beating yourself down with negative thoughts and hateful discourse, learn how to be compassionate with yourself.

At the beginning of my healing process, I was angry at myself; I didn't want to make peace with the fact that I let someone treat me like that. I felt foolish and naive, and this made it more difficult for me to love myself. Through patience and time, I found a way to forgive myself for my past mistakes, and I looked at my past wounded self with compassion. I understood that I was only trying to heal unresolved wounds from my past, and I just didn't know any better. What mattered was that I got myself out of that situation, and I started working on creating a better life for myself.

To find inner peace, not only did I have to learn how to be compassionate with myself, but I had to find a way to forgive the narcissist. However, this time my forgiveness was different. I didn't forgive his abusive behavior to take him back. I didn't forgive him for how much he hurt me, to find a way to stay in the relationship. I forgave him because I didn't want to stay stuck with feelings of anger and resentment. I wanted to be completely free and start a new chapter in my life filled with feelings of positivity, joy, love, and peace.

Spend Time with Your Tribe

Connecting with others who have similar interests helps you cultivate a sense of belonging. You feel inspired and get new ideas that enrich your life. Hanging with your kind of people makes you feel joyful and uplifted. If you're not sure where you can meet your tribe, start going to places and events which genuinely interest you, and you'll naturally find them there. For example, if you like art, you can visit museums and gallery exhibitions, if you like history or food, go on a tour, and you'll surely bump into someone and naturally start a conversation. If you enjoy reading, you can join a book club; they can be really fun!

After being surrounded by someone who used to consistently bring me down, it was truly refreshing to spend time with people who helped me feel good about life in general. I had forgotten how it felt to spend time with people who don't make you feel like you want to stop breathing as they're speaking to you. Try it out and surround yourself with people who love you and respect you for who you are. Relax and enjoy being in their presence.

I'd like to close this chapter by emphasizing that falling in love with yourself is a process. It's also a choice, one that you will have to make again and again. Just like in any relationship, there will be moments when you fall off track, when you regress into old patterns, or when self-doubt creeps in. And that's okay. The key is to be mindful of it and, when you notice yourself slipping into self-destructive tendencies, always return to self-compassion.

Shaming or judging yourself will only pull you deeper into a spiral of negativity. And I say this from experience—patterns can be incredibly strong. I like to think of them as a blueprint, an algorithm, much like a computer program running on its existing code. To change that program, you have to rewrite the code, and that takes time, effort, and conscious awareness. Change is never instant, but it is always possible.

Even after doing deep inner healing, I've found that specific triggers can still bring out my old self. But the difference is that as you become more conscious and self-aware, you're able to catch yourself faster. And that awareness gives you a powerful choice. It doesn't matter how many times you fall back into old habits. What truly matters is that you pick yourself up and keep moving forward from where you left off.

So let this be your reminder to be gentle and kind to yourself. Falling in love with yourself is a lifelong journey—one of peeling back the layers, discovering more about who you are, embracing the things you love about yourself, and learning to accept the things you don't. And that's okay! Love every part of you, even the ones that feel dark or shameful. Because only by acknowledging and embracing them can you integrate, transmute, and free yourself from their grip.

- **INSIGHTFUL LESSON:** Falling in love with yourself is a choice you will make again and again. When you stray from it, guide yourself back with kindness, and compassion. Always return to love.

Chapter 19

Breaking the Habit of Bad Relationships

ONE PARTICULAR EVENING, THE narcissist and I had gone for dinner at a restaurant. We ordered our food, but within minutes, a heated argument erupted. Our fights were so frequent that I don't even remember what this one was about. What I do remember is that we had been arguing for hours, so caught up in the conflict that we failed to notice the waiters had completely forgotten our order.

Lost in the argument, we lost all sense of time. Neither of us was aware of our surroundings until a sudden noise and commotion in the background snapped us out of it. Only then did we look around and realize that the restaurant was closing—and our food had never even been served.

This experience was a wake-up call. I was shocked at how unaware I was of what was happening around me. Not only did I lose track of time and spend over 3 hours arguing without noticing that the food hadn't been served, but I didn't even realize that all the people had left, that my heart was racing, and that I was shaking with anger and frustration. I started reflecting on my life and realized that, most of the time, I wasn't mentally present—not in my daily experiences, nor in my interactions with others. My mind was always wandering, obsessing over the relationship, stressing over his moods, or replaying past arguments. I lived on autopilot, constantly acting impulsively and reacting emotionally to triggers. I was living in a mindless state—the complete opposite of mindfulness. No wonder I was constantly losing things, forgetting details, and feeling completely scattered.

Grace is describing both a hypervigilant and a dissociated state. Living with the narcissist put her in constant fight-flight-fawn reactiveness; she existed with an activated sympathetic nervous system, which is when you are on high alert because you feel that you are in danger—what I identify as code yellow, orange, or red. We are scanning the environment, we are bug-eyed, we can never relax, not even when asleep, and we are unable to be aware of anything else because peril is at hand.

It makes perfect sense for our bodies to go into a hypervigilant state—and in fact, we are thankful that it knows to sound the alarms of danger in order to help us find safety—but when it becomes the norm, as in cases of war and abuse, our systems are memorizing trauma and being flooded with cortisol showers, the stress hormone. Forgetfulness, "spacing out," freezing, inability to sleep, and impulsiveness are all symptoms of trauma and post-traumatic stress. General anxiety disorder and ADHD share the same symptoms and can sometimes be the cover story for deeply buried trauma. Love does not exist here, only fear.

When your body is in survival mode due to abuse, and when you're constantly in fight or flight mode, it means that your limbic system is overactive, which surely makes it more difficult to think clearly and be mindful. Luckily, the brain is an adaptive organ, and we can rewire the neural pathways in our brains through certain mindfulness exercises. Dr. Joe Dispenza has done extensive work on neuroplasticity, the brain's ability to rewire and adapt through conscious effort and practice. Before we explore the mindfulness exercises that you can explore, it's important to understand what mindfulness actually is and why it has the power to change your life.

As I briefly explained earlier, neuroplasticity is a neuroscientific finding that demonstrates the brain's ability to continue growing and forming new synaptic connections, even after an injury, and I would add, even after trauma. I call neuroplasticity the HOPE DISCOVERY because it has provided hope for millions! Neuroplasticity basically says that even when we have had a brain injury, even when we have been to war, even when we have an abusive childhood, and even after we have been in a relationship with a narcissist, our brain can expand into new healing. But this is the clincher...how does it do that?

Answer: Through having new experiences! Isn't this amazing? Picture an enlaced web of connections. These connections or neuroassociations (remember "the more we fire, the more we wire") can multiply into more connections by having new experiences. New experiences can include the unconditional regard of a coach, a strong and nurturing relationship with a therapist, a physical setting that feels consistently safe, and so on. By having new and caring experiences, the brain can "stretch" beyond the injury/trauma and literally form a new neural net that includes safety and secure attachment.

Can you see why I call neuroplasticity the hope discovery?! So mindfulness fits in perfectly here. If having a secure attached relationship with someone is an INTERpersonal new experience, mindfulness meditation is an INTRApersonal new experience where we have a kind and loving relationship with ourselves. It massively counts towards neuroplasticity!

Here's how some of the most influential mindfulness teachers define it:

- **Eckhart Tolle**, author of *The Power of Now*, highlights mindfulness as the act of being fully present, observing our thoughts and emotions without getting caught up in them, leading to a profound sense of inner peace.

- **Jack Kornfield**, a renowned mindfulness teacher and former Buddhist monk, emphasizes that mindfulness is about being present with kindness and openness, cultivating a deep connection with ourselves and the world around us.

- **Tara Brach**, a leading meditation teacher and psychologist, describes mindfulness as paying attention to our inner life with curiosity and compassion, allowing us to embrace our true selves.

These teachings have been deeply influential in my personal mindfulness journey, and I feel incredibly grateful to be training under Jack Kornfield and Tara Brach in my mindfulness teacher program. Their wisdom has helped me understand the transformative power of meeting ourselves with kindness and compassion. By integrating these perspectives, we can see that mindfulness is about cultivating self-awareness in a way that empowers us to make conscious choices rather than reacting impulsively, leading to a more balanced and fulfilling life.

Why Mindfulness Matters in Healing

Mindfulness ultimately gives you power over your actions. So, the next time the narcissist texts you asking to meet up or get back together, you won't act on impulse—instead, you'll be able to pause, reflect, and respond consciously, rather than letting emotions take over.

Remember the 4 Ps: pause which gives you power which gives you possibility which gives you prowess. You become a new person through your new responses to people, places, and things. You trust yourself, a sublime arrival point.

According to the YMCA of Greater Brandywine's website (n.d.), mindfulness can be utilized to rewire the brain ("Using Mindfulness to Rewire Your Brain"). This process is similar to rewriting a computer program's code, as I explained in the previous chapter—by making these internal changes, you can start creating different outcomes in your life.

Practicing mindfulness creates space between your thoughts and yourself. You become less identified with them, and therefore you take the seat of the observer. When this shift occurs, it allows you to take a step back and examine the relationship with greater clarity, enabling you to understand what was truly happening. So I started questioning why I acted in certain ways, why I tolerated the abuse, and I slowly started having more control over my actions and choices. Mindfulness helped me reclaim my power. It was the main tool that helped me transform from a naive powerless victim of manipulation and gaslighting, to the person I am today.

Yes! Grace embodied the 4 Ps!

The more I practiced mindfulness meditation, the more I was able to live in the present moment and see the beauty in it. I freed myself from the mental prison that I was living in by detaching from negative thoughts and heavy emotions that were disturbing my peace. As the saying goes, knowledge is power, and when you gain self-knowledge, you have the power in your hands to change the direction of your life.

Grace's description of gaining power through self-knowledge is what I promote as getting a PhD on yourSELF. When we know a topic thoroughly, like when we get a doctorate on it, we become a well-versed expert, and so why not get a PhD on yourSELF? Notice that as she did this, her central nervous system came back to baseline, and activated the parasympathetic system, defined as the "rest and digest" state. It is called this because in a calm, functioning state, we can relax, sleep, and eat because we feel safe. When the opposite is activated, the sympathetic system, we are preparing for danger, with quick shallow breaths, blood rushing towards the limbs away from the digestive region, because when we feel in danger, we are prepared to fight or flee from it. Mindfulness meditation which helps in quieting the mind and slowing down breathing can put us in a parasympathetic state.

Cultivating Mindfulness

There are many ways to practice mindfulness. While meditation is a powerful tool, it's just one form of mindfulness practice. You don't have to meditate for hours like a monk to reap its benefits. Mindfulness can be practiced in small, intentional moments throughout your day.

Scientific research has shown that mindfulness practices, particularly meditation, can significantly reduce stress, enhance focus, and improve emotional well-being. Studies have even demonstrated that regular meditation rewires the brain, strengthening areas associated with self-awareness, emotional regulation, and resilience (American Psychological Association, n.d.).

That being said, you don't have to force yourself into meditation if it doesn't feel right for you. Mindfulness comes in many forms, and I encourage you to explore different practices until you find what works best. Below, I share some approaches that have helped me in my own journey toward self-awareness.

Mindfulness Meditation Practice

Incorporating mindfulness meditation into your daily routine can be as simple as brushing your teeth every morning and night. Start with just 5 minutes in the morning before you begin your day, and 5 minutes before going to sleep. As you get more comfortable, you can gradually extend your practice.

To help make it a habit, link meditation to something you already do daily. Maybe you meditate right after waking up or right before bed, as long as you stay awake and engaged. The goal isn't to do it because you "have to" but because you want to—because you want to become more present, take better care of yourself, and strengthen your mind.

Think of meditation like a mental workout. Every time your mind wanders and you gently bring it back to your breath, you're strengthening your focus, just like lifting a weight builds muscle.

I encourage you to look into the scientific research behind meditation and its countless benefits. It has been shown to improve mental clarity, emotional regulation, and even physical health. But at its core, allowing yourself to take the meditation seat is an act of radical self-love!

Walk Mindfully in Nature

Spending time in nature has been scientifically proven to reduce stress and anxiety while enhancing overall well-being. Nature has a unique healing energy, and learning how to immerse yourself in it truly can help you raise your vibrational frequency.

One way to practice mindfulness is by engaging all your senses while walking in nature:

- **Sight:** Observe the landscape, the colors, the way sunlight filters through the trees, or the movement of water.
- **Hearing:** Listen to the sounds of birds chirping, the rustling leaves, or the waves crashing against the shore.
- **Touch:** Feel the breeze on your skin, the warmth of the sun, or the cool earth beneath your feet.
- **Smell:** Notice the scent of fresh rain on the soil, the salty ocean breeze, or the fragrance of flowers around you.

By focusing on the present moment, you can quiet your mind and reconnect with yourself through nature's grounding energy.

Mindful Conversations

The next time you have a conversation with someone or find yourself in a meeting at work, make an intentional effort to focus and listen attentively. We're all guilty of drifting off in thought during conversations, but practicing mindful listening helps you get out of your head and be more present with whoever you are with.

Mindful listening also helps us to listen without judgment. Often, while someone is speaking, we're already formulating our response in our heads before they've even finished. Instead, try to be fully present. Listen with empathy and focus on understanding rather than preparing what you're going to say next.

And when it's your turn to speak, be mindful of your words. Take a moment to pause and reflect on what you truly want to express. Speak with intention, clarity, and kindness. Mindful speaking is just as important as mindful listening. It fosters open and honest communication, helping to create deeper, more meaningful connections.

You'll be amazed at how much this simple shift can improve your communication skills and open you up to new perspectives. Our judgments and assumptions limit our understanding, but listening without judgment and speaking with presence creates space for genuine connection and insight.

Music Meditation & Mindful Movement

Music meditation combined with mindful movement is a powerful practice that helps you connect more deeply with your body, emotions, and spirit. It's an intuitive and liberating way to process emotions, release stored tension, and feel more alive and present in your body.

This practice can be as straightforward or as profound as you allow it to be. You don't need to be a dancer, and it's not about moving in any particular way. It's about tuning in and letting your body lead. You may find yourself swaying gently, stretching, or moving with wild, expressive freedom. There's no right or wrong, only what feels authentic in the moment.

Here's how you can try it:

1. Find a space where you feel safe and comfortable, free from distractions or the fear of being observed.
2. Put on a pair of headphones, if possible (though it's not necessary), so you can fully immerse yourself in the music. Choose music that resonates with you—whether calming, energizing, or emotional.
3. Close your eyes if it feels right and take a few deep breaths to ground yourself. As the music plays, focus all your attention on the sounds and how they make you feel.

4. Notice if the music stirs something within you. Without overthinking it, allow your body to move in response to the rhythm and melody. Don't worry about how you look or whether it makes sense. Let it be raw, real, and intuitive.

This practice reconnects you to your body's innate wisdom and can be incredibly healing. As you move, you may notice emotions rising—whether joy, sadness, or release. Let it all move through you. The act of mindful movement helps you process and express feelings that may have been trapped inside, offering a sense of freedom and emotional release. Ultimately, living mindfully improves every aspect of your life, from the relationship with yourself to your relationships with others. Mindfulness helps you become aware of your needs, thought processes, and emotions, and it helps you understand yourself at a deeper level. It is a tool that helps you quiet the ego and open the door to your true essence to shine its light. With some patience, practice, and commitment, everyone can learn how to develop this skill, and it can truly be beneficial not only in your healing process but throughout the rest of your life.

Chapter 20

Shadow Work & The Power of Mindset

WE ARE ALL SHAPED by invisible forces we rarely question and are mostly unaware of. Some are etched in our DNA, passed down through generations, while others are molded by the environments we grow up in and the experiences we endure. Both nature and nurture work together to create the beliefs, behaviors, and patterns that govern our lives, whether we're aware of them or not.

Looking back, I can clearly see how I was a product of both. I inherited deeply ingrained tendencies toward codependency and people-pleasing from my family, and my early experiences only reinforced these patterns. I was molded into someone who felt responsible for other people's happiness.

What I've come to understand is that, beyond our personal history, we also carry archetypal patterns within us. These are universal roles and themes that play out across cultures and generations. I had been unconsciously embodying the archetype of the Caregiver and the Rescuer, constantly giving to others at the expense of myself, believing it was my duty to save, fix, or heal those around me. These patterns were so familiar, they felt like second nature. But they also kept me stuck in unhealthy dynamics where my worth was tied to what I could offer others, not who I was at my core.

At the time, I had no idea that my subconscious programming and these archetypal roles I had been playing were responsible for the hellish relationship I found myself in. I thought I was just unlucky in love, or maybe not good enough to be treated well. What I didn't realize was that I was running an old mental program, a blueprint shaped by years of conditioning and unconscious archetypes that kept pulling me toward the same painful experiences on repeat.

We remember interchangeable phrases such as mental models, psychological patterns, relational schemas, neuro associations, or neural nets, and attachment styles. They all represent a similar idea, which is that we have internalized patterns of relating that were learned during our childhood from our families of origin, our culture, our religion, and even our ancestry.

In Dynamic, I call this "the sleeping volcano" because they lie dormant until we trigger them into a not-so-pretty explosion. These unconscious knots form into a swell of reactivity when they run up against our external life. Most of the time, these are unconscious until we make them conscious through self-reflection and analysis. A good phrase or healing mantra that I use is "thank you triggers because you lead me to the fault lines that lead me to the goldmines." Neuroplasticity is the process of alchemizing the faultiness into goldmines, and it tells us that we can form a new mindset through our conscious work.

But how do we break free from these unconscious patterns?

This is where shadow work becomes essential. Shadow work is the process of exploring the hidden parts of yourself—the subconscious beliefs, wounds, and patterns that influence your thoughts, emotions, and actions without you even realizing it. Psychiatrist Carl Jung described the shadow as the "unknown dark side of the personality." He famously said: "Until you make the unconscious conscious, it will direct your life and you will call it fate."

Shadow work invites you to meet these hidden parts with compassion and curiosity, rather than fear, shame, or judgment. When you bring light to your shadows, you reclaim your power. You integrate what you once rejected or disowned, becoming more whole and authentic. This is how you free yourself from outdated subconscious programming and step into your full potential.

For me, shadow work was a turning point. As I began to uncover the unconscious beliefs and wounded parts that had shaped my identity and behavior, I realized I had the power to choose differently. I no longer had to play the same roles or live out the same painful cycles. As we learned in the previous chapter, mindfulness is a powerful tool that helps us become more conscious. It gives us the awareness and clarity we need to recognize these old patterns as they arise, allowing us to make better choices and create a better life for ourselves.

Shadow work can be approached in various ways, and it's often best to start with the guidance of a skilled professional, such as a trauma-informed therapist, somatic practitioner, or shadow work coach. Some approaches include guided inner child healing, parts work (like Internal Family Systems therapy), somatic shadow work, or journaling prompts that help you explore hidden emotions and beliefs. Practices like breathwork, meditation, and somatic therapy can also help you access and integrate these deeper layers of yourself.

As you do this deep inner work, pairing it with mindset reprogramming makes the transformation even more powerful. Through practices like mindfulness, cognitive reframing, and the principles of neuroplasticity, you can begin to rewrite the mental programs that have been running your life. This combination of shadow work and mindset work creates lasting change. You're not just becoming aware of old patterns;

you're consciously choosing new ones and reinforcing them, creating a new, empowered blueprint for your life.

So what is "*mindset*?" A mindset is a set of beliefs, attitudes, and behaviors that shapes our reality. It's our mental program that runs the show, and most often, we are unaware of the beliefs and attitudes that dictate our lives. Let's have a look at some typical mindsets that keep us stuck in toxic relationships:

Taking Things Personally

When I was still in the relationship, I used to internalize everything that went wrong. The fact that the narcissist used to blame me for everything surely didn't help. However, the fact that I took things personally reflected how insecure I felt about myself. When you really know your self-worth, you won't let anyone affect how you feel about yourself. Now that I've learned my true value, I understand that his attitude and approach towards adverse situations had nothing to do with me, but were a reflection of who he is as a person.

By not taking things personally, Grace is also describing no longer feeling codependent. His opinions, judgments, and criticisms were no longer entangled with her sovereign sense of herself. A good time to use one of my Claudisms, or phrases that I use to emotionally calibrate, mentally reframe, and spiritually connect with the now moment: "Your story is not my story."

Fixer Mentality

I was the kind of person who felt responsible for other people's feelings, especially when it came to pain and discomfort. I felt an intense need to help others feel better, even if it meant neglecting myself in the process. Teaching myself that everyone is responsible for their own feelings helped me free myself from trying to protect the narcissist and make sure that he was okay. I also freed myself from the responsibility of trying to fix the relationship against all odds. If something or someone is endangering my well-being, my responsibility is to protect myself and make sure that I'm okay.

Moving away from saving and fixing also moves Grace from being a wounded Empath to a healed, empowered Empath! Even though she can still feel things and people deeply, she does not have to take on their suffering, trauma, and even better, she is not enslaved to saving them. Remember, the Empath automatically tries to harmonize environments so that they can feel better, an impossible feat when living in a trauma world. She can now regulate herself, harmonize her own internal experience through mindfulness and boundaries, without having to fix anything outside of herself. Champagne bottles popping!

Over-Idealizing

From the moment I met the narcissist, I had put him on a pedestal. I felt like a 5-year-old girl in a fairy tale being saved by her knight in shining armor. It's clear to me now that I was unconsciously embodying the Wounded Child archetype. That part of me was still longing to be rescued, to be loved unconditionally, and to finally feel safe in someone else's care. When you over-idealize someone, it means that you are forgetting your self-worth and how valuable you are. It means that you feel unworthy and undeserving of this person. Later on, I learned that to have a healthy relationship, you need to both feel equally worthy of each other, so you have a balance of power in the relationship.

When we are wounded and recovering from neglect, abandonment, and trauma, it truly feels like the other person who chooses to love us is the answer to everything. We can feel like we just won the relationship lottery because they are willing to love us. It's quite painful even to describe this level of internal loneliness and low self-worth. No child or person should feel so unloved that someone choosing to love them automatically establishes a massive power imbalance.

We can clearly see why a neglected child might easily succumb to the advances of a sexual predator just to get love, and possibly even idealize them as a loving caregiver. Idealization and emotional molestation can go hand in hand. Placing them on a pedestal feels accurate because they feel superior, and any crumbs of attention feel like a windfall. Equality between partners, or humans, can exist when both are seen as sovereign beings and mutually respected as such.

Acknowledging that I was a victim of domestic violence was an important step in my healing journey. Denying what happened wouldn't have gotten me anywhere. However, if I stayed stuck in self-narrative stories of self-pity and despair, I would have stayed like that—a victim. If you get stuck in this state, it means that you are keeping yourself in a vulnerable position. This can only attract more predators into your life who are ready to take advantage of you. Moving forward and cultivating a resilient mindset helps you transform yourself from victim to survivor to warrior.

Ask yourself if being a victim is a persona that got you attention? Ask yourself if victimhood feels self-soothing because you can nurse old wounds over and over? Notice if being a victim truly gets you what you truly want. It is unlikely. As Grace states, it will, however, repeat the same cycle of abuse over and over. A victim requires an abuser and a savior. The victim-savior-aggressor paradigm is at the center of all codependency and toxic relationships across the board, including systemic, cultural, and ancestral ones.

Negative Mindset

When you're going through a difficult period in your life, it's easy to focus on negativity, and you might struggle to see the light. The more you focus on what's going wrong in your life, the harder it will be for you to lift yourself up and create a positive change. Step by step, you can train your mind to focus on the positive things in life and be grateful for all that you have, no matter how small or insignificant they might seem to you at the time. Shifting to a positive mindset allowed me to create powerful shifts and transformations in my life.

A good motivation for changing a negative mindset is the concept of the perceptual field. What we hold in mind only grows. If you have negative thinking, you will only see the negative in life because of that very narrow perceptual field. It creates a self-fulfilling prophecy that at first you can allocate to another, but once you become conscious of it, you can take the wheel of where your attention goes. This is not an easy endeavor, but again, a worthy one. As Grace asked in an earlier chapter, and I paraphrase, all of this is hard, but which hard will you choose? The hard of being abused or the hard of doing the healing work?

Locus of Control

Throughout my relationship, I was always trying to control the narcissist and external situations. It was exhausting trying to prevent him from cheating, keeping an eye on his every move, and trying to keep it together. No matter how hard I tried, I still didn't manage to control anything. He still cheated whenever he wanted, and things still got out of hand. If anything, I made things worse by trying to control them. What I learned from this experience is that the only thing we have control over is ourselves. This helped me take responsibility for my actions, and I learned how to master my own energy to create the life that I wanted.

I love the term "locus of control"! It is a very psychological word used often when psychotherapists analyze their patients. Where is the person's locus of control? Inside themselves or outside of themselves? The journey from shifting the locus of control from external to internal is a long one, but it is precisely the objective of the psychological and spiritual journey. We learn that peace comes from within, so does love, strength, worthiness, and so on. When we can anchor into a strong internal locus of control, we are smack in the middle of our higher Self. It is a strong marker of having moved from trauma surviving to trauma rising. Ah, locus of control! What empowering, beautiful words!

Expecting Others to Complete You

Many of us make the mistake of waiting for someone to make us feel whole and complete. We fail to realize that we are already whole, and that anyone who comes into our lives is a bonus. This kind of mindset immediately puts you in an inferior position. It implies that you need someone else to feel happy in your life. You end up expecting others to fulfill your needs and make you feel good and joyful.

Yes, the concept of "you complete me," a trendy phrase to describe romantic love, is actually more of a sign of codependency and low self-worth. Compassion is essential here. The person who has never been seen, heard, or validated truly feels invisible, as if they don't exist, as if they are nothing. When someone appears in their life and sees them, even details like the narcissist does, it is hard not to feel like they are completing you, as if they are filling the perimeter inside you with a crayon. To be seen, witnessed, or beamed at is a human treasure.

Sadly, when this happens through the gaze of abuse, it is destruction. So, rather, look in the mirror. Look at yourSELF over and over and say "I love you" and "I complete me." Find coaches, therapists, groups, and friends who will gaze at you and help you see that you are whole. We are reminded of Lester Levinson, "When the love is complete, the problem is solved." Indeed. You complete you with your own love.

We don't realize how we are placing our happiness in someone else's hands, and that we are completely giving away our power. Realizing that I was responsible for my own happiness was an eye opener, and it gave me the power to create a life that I loved.

INSIGHTFUL LESSON: Unlearn what you have learned and set yourself free!

FINAL THOUGHTS

EVERYONE'S HEALING JOURNEY IS different. What's important is that you put into practice what you've learned from this book and from any other sources you've found helpful along the way. Don't be too hard on yourself; everyone has setbacks. What matters most is that you pick yourself up again and keep moving forward.

Don't underestimate your own personal power and capabilities. We discover our strength when life tests us. Connecting to a greater power beyond the physical world has been the driving force that helped me move mountains and overcome what I once thought I would never be able to.

Have faith in yourself. Trust that everything will be okay—and it will be when you start doing the inner work. Something beautiful awaits you on the other side of your healing journey. Listen to your heart and let it guide you. Heal your wounds through self-love and acceptance. Let your light shine through your deepest wounds, and allow your most beautiful, authentic self to emerge.

Wishing you Peace, Love, and Light,

—Grace

I BELIEVE THAT WE CAN heal through secure adult attachment bonds. When we feel securely attached, we feel, first and foremost, safe. Safety comes in many forms, and one of them is feeling like our parents, our guides, or the person who knows more than we do—even if it's a few steps more—provides us with information, instructions, and a roadmap, all enveloped in love and patience. This bedrock of safety becomes the launchpad for exploration, expansion, and evolution. In this book, Grace has done this beautifully! You are about to embark on a journey of self-discovery because she has provided the roadmap, the instructions, and the caring resonance you will need to explore deep parts of yourself.

—Claudia

ABOUT THE AUTHORS

Grace Being began sharing the mindfulness techniques that helped her break away from toxic patterns after healing from her own experience with narcissistic abuse. Alongside her mindfulness work, Grace embraces song as a form of expression, using music to spread joy, inspire creativity, and connect with people. She currently leads mindfulness sessions in Valencia, Spain, and offers an online recovery program for those struggling with narcissistic abuse.

Claudia Cauterucci, LPC is an internationally recognized psychotherapist, intuitive speaker, and trauma-informed thought leader. She is the visionary behind the Dynamic Meditation Healing Modality and the Dynamic R-Evolution Movement, pioneering approaches that integrate emotional intelligence, somatic healing, and spiritual insight. Claudia is the author of *The Empath Leader*, a groundbreaking guide that redefines leadership through the lens of empathy and resilience. Based in Washington, D.C., Claudia leads a thriving therapy practice and facilitates The Empath Leader, a transformative 12-week leadership training designed for C-suite executives, creatives, and influencers. Developed in response to post-pandemic socio-political shifts, the program elevates the role of the empath as a catalyst for conscious change. She also hosts and produces the podcast Heaven on Earth, where she spotlights visionary guests who are cultivating intimacy, healing, and dynamic solutions for a more harmonious world.

REFERENCES

PsychCentral. (2013, July 6). Narcissists' Lack of Empathy Tied to Less Gray Matter. Retrieved from https://psychcentral.com/news/2013/07/06/narcissists-lack-of-empathy-tied-to-less-gray-matter

Mayo Clinic. (n.d.). Narcissistic Personality Disorder. Retrieved from https://www.mayoclinic.org/diseases-conditions/narcissistic-personality-disorder/symptoms-causes/syc-20366662

NeuroInstincts. (n.d.). Idealize, Devalue, Discard: The Dizzying Cycle of Narcissism. Retrieved from https://neuroinstincts.com/idealize-devalue-discard/

PsychCentral. (n.d.). Denial of Trauma Signs: How to Know If Someone Is in Denial. Retrieved from https://psychcentral.com/blog/denial-of-trauma-signs#how-to-know-someones-in-denial

American Psychological Association. (2014). Chronic Stress. Retrieved from https://www.apa.org/monitor/2014/10/chronic-stress

EFT International. (n.d.). What is EFT Tapping? Retrieved from https://eftinternational.org/discover-eft-tapping/what-is-eft-tapping/

MentalHelp.net. (n.d.). Emotional and Social Development and Understanding. Retrieved from https://www.mentalhelp.net/infancy/emotional-social-development-and-understanding/

Child Welfare Information Gateway. (n.d.). The Impact of Trauma on Child Brain Development and Behavior [PDF document]. Retrieved from https://www.childwelfare.gov/pubpdfs/braindevtrauma.pdf

Practice Notes. (n.d.). Understanding the Effects of Maltreatment on Brain Development. Retrieved from https://practicenotes.org/v17n2/brain.htm

Goleman, D. (n.d.). Research Supports SEL. Edutopia. Retrieved from https://www.edutopia.org/blog/daniel-goleman-research-supports-sel-betty-ray

Timothy T. Brown and Terry L. Jernigan (2012). Brain development during the preschool years. NCBI, Article PMC351163) https://www.ncbi.nlm.nih.gov/pmc/articles/PMC3511633/

University of Washington. (2006, September 12). Violence in the Home Leads to Higher Rates of Childhood Bullying. Retrieved from https://www.washington.edu/news/2006/09/12/violence-in-the-home-leads-to-higher-rates-of-childhood-bullying/

Can Narcissism Be Cured, Psych Central. Retrieved from https://psychcentral.com/disorders/narcissistic-personality-disorder/narcissism-cure#cure-for-narcissism

John Bowlby and Mary Ainsworth. (1992). The origins of attachment theory: APA PsycNET. Retrieved from https://psycnet.apa.org/record/1993-01038-001

PsychCentral (2019, March 31). Narcissists Use Trauma Bonding and Intermittent Reinforcement To Get You Addicted To Them: Why Abuse Survivors Stay. Psych Central. Retrieved from https://psychcentral.com/blog/recovering-narcissist/2019/03/narcissists-use-trauma-bonding-and-intermittent-reinforcement-to-get-you-addicted-to-them-why-abuse-survivors-stay

Harvard Health Publishing. (n.d.). What is somatic therapy? Harvard Health Blog. Retrieved from https://www.health.harvard.edu/blog/what-is-somatic-therapy-202307072951

American Psychological Association. (n.d.). Meditation and mindfulness. Retrieved from https://www.apa.org/topics/mindfulness/meditation

News18. (n.d.). Survey Identifies 'Self-Love Crisis' Around the World. Retrieved from https://www.news18.com/news/lifestyle/survey-identifies-self-love-crisis-around-the-world-3521621.html

Dr. Joe Dispenza. (n.d.). Unlimited Dr Joe Dispenza. Retrieved from https://drjoedispenza.com/blogs/dr-joes-blog/can-you-change-your-brain-by-thinking-differently

YMCA of Greater BrandyWine. (n.d.). YMCA For Youth Development, Healthy Living, and Social Responsibility. Retrieved from https://ymcagbw.org/blog/using-mindfulness-rewire-your-brain